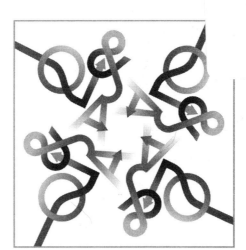

Blueprints

STEP 1
Q & A

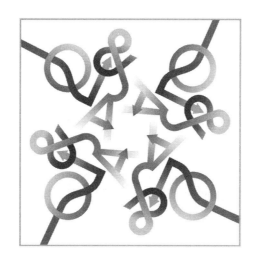

Blueprints

STEP 1
Q & A

EDITOR:

Michael S. Clement, MD, FAAP

Mountain Park Health Center, Phoenix, Arizona

Clinical Lecturer in Family and Community Medicine
University of Arizona College of Medicine

Consultant, Arizona Department of Health Services

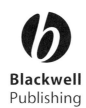

Blackwell
Publishing

Blackwell Publishing, Inc.
   350 Main Street, Malden, Massachusetts 02148-5018, USA
Blackwell Publishing Ltd
   9600 Garsington Road, Oxford OX4 2DQ, UK
Blackwell Science Asia Pty Ltd
   550 Swanston Street, Carlton, Victoria 3053, Australia
Blackwell Verlag GmbH, Kurfürstendamm 57, 10707 Berlin, Germany

02 03 04 05 5 4 3 2 1

ISBN: 1-4051-0323-X

Library of Congress Cataloging-in-Publication Data

Blueprints step 1 Q&A / editor, Michael S. Clement.
      p. ; cm. — (Blueprints)
   ISBN 1-40510-323-X (pbk.)
   1. Medicine — Examinations, questions, etc. 2. Clinical
medicine — Examinations, questions, etc.
   [DNLM: 1. Clinical Medicine--Examination Questions. WB 18.2 B6584
2003] I. Title: Blueprints step 1 Q&A. II. Title: Blueprints step one
Q&A. III. Clement, Michael S. IV. Series.

R834.5 .B583 2003
616'.0076--dc21   2002015311

A catalogue record for this title is available from the British Library

Acquisitions: Beverly Copland
Development: Julia Casson/William Deluise
Production: Jennifer Kowalewski
Cover design: Hannus Design Associates
Interior design: Leslie Haimes
Typesetter: International Typesetting and Composition, in India
Printed and bound by Malloy Lithographing, Inc., in Michigan

For further information on Blackwell Publishing, visit our website:
www.medirect.com

NOTICE: The indications and dosages of all drugs in this book have been recommended in the medical literature and conform to the practices of the general community. The
medications described and treatment prescriptions suggested do not necessarily have
specific approval by the Food and Drug Administration for use in the diseases and
dosages for which they are recommended. The package insert for each drug should be
consulted for use and dosage as approved by the FDA. Because standards for usage
change, it is advisable to keep abreast of revised recommendations, particularly those
concerning new drugs.

TABLE OF CONTENTS

PREFACE

You've worked and studied hard for two years, and now it's time for the USMLE Step 1. What you need now are lots of clinical questions to practice.

Blueprints *Step 1 Q & A* was developed *Just For You!* Medical students who recently took the exam wrote these questions to help other students know *what to study*. The questions and answers were then reviewed by other medical students to ensure the accuracy and quality.

Blueprints *Step 1 Q & A* is a complete length exam that simulates the real one. Study one block in 50 minutes, when you have time. Or, practice a day of testing, just like the exam, by timing each block as you go.

You'll find this new review book offers just what you are looking for, including:

• Full-length practice exam of 350 questions
• Written by students who recently took the exam
• Questions integrated in blocks of 50, just like the exam
• Short concise answers with rationales for all options
• Clinical cases replicate the USMLE format
• Board format questions with **no "except" questions**
• All **new** questions

Get the practice you need—and be confident when you take the exam.

All of the authors and staff at Blackwell wish you well on the Boards and in your medical future. We welcome feedback and suggestions you may have about this book. Send comments to blue@blacksci.com.

CONTRIBUTORS

Shanti Lal Bansal
Class of 2004
Rush Medical College, Chicago, Illinois

Shanti is currently a second-year medical student at Rush Medical College, Chicago. He earned a bachelor of science degree at Johns Hopkins University in both computer science and biomedical engineering. Shanti is well published in the field of orthopedic surgery. He was born in New Delhi, India, and grew up in New Hampshire.

Amy Connell
Class of 2000
University of Iowa, Iowa City, Iowa

Amy is currently in her second year of psychiatry residency at the University of Wisconsin in Madison. She received her medical degree from the University of Iowa. When she's not working, Amy enjoys spending time with her black lab, Wally, and running and is planning for her first marathon in June 2002.

Michael T. Czarnecki
Class of 2003
Ross University School of Medicine, New York City, New York

Michael is a graduate of the United States Air Force Military Academy and is now a fourth year medical student in New York City. Before starting his pursuit of an MD degree, Michael served as an officer in the U.S. Air Force, with service across the world as an explosives engineer. Michael holds a degree in mechanical engineering and further pursued becoming an EMT-P, NREMT-P, and CCEMT-P while in the Air Force. He is the author of the Critical Care Transport Field Guide as well as contributing editor to the Critical Care Transport Textbook. Along with being well published in the field of emergency medicine, Michael is a visiting instructor at the University of Maryland, Baltimore Campus Emergency Health Services paramedic program. He looks forward to a residency position in Emergency Medicine or Critical Care Medicine.

Mila Felder
Class of 2002
Chicago Medical School, North Chicago, Illinois

Mila did her undergraduate work in applied mathematics at Odessa State University in Odessa, Ukraine. Her active academic and professional life since arriving to the United States in 1991 includes studying at California State University, Los Angeles, and managing a busy medical practice, and then initiation and management of a surgical center. Inspired by doctors she worked with, she proceeded to medical school.

She received her masters of science in physiology and a medical degree from Chicago Medical School, where she graduated at the top 20% of her class and is now entering an emergency medicine residency program at Christ Hospital in Oak Lawn, IL. Her husband, a computer programmer, and her son, a very devoted hockey player (he is turning 9 this summer), have always been a great support and a driving force for Mila's inspiration and persistence at accomplishing her dream of obtaining a medical degree.

James Fletcher
Class of 2003
Eastern Virginia Medical School, Norfolk, Virginia

James received his BA in history from the University of Virginia in 1992 and then went on to earn a doctor of podiatric medicine degree from the Ohio College of Podiatric Medicine in 1997. He is currently a Naval Reserve Officer with the HPSP program at Eastern Virginia Medical School.

Jonathan Gottlieb
Class of 2002
University of Miami, Miami, Florida

Jonathan graduated from the University of Miami School of Medicine in 2002 and is now an orthopaedic surgery resident at Jackson Memorial Hospital in Miami, FL. He is interested in pursuing a spine surgery fellowship and is currently involved in various research projects regarding spinal injuries and surgeries.

Christopher Hughes
Class of 2003
Texas Tech University Health Sciences Center
 School of Medicine, El Paso, Texas

Christopher received a bachelor of science degree in biology from the University of Texas at Arlington in 1997 and worked for two years doing research at the University of Texas Southwestern Medical Center before entering medical school in 1999. Upon graduation he intends to complete a residency in pediatrics.

Brendan Kelley
Class of 2002
Ohio State University, Columbus, Ohio

Brendan attended the Ohio State University for undergraduate study, graduating with a B.S. in physics and a B.A. in Russian literature. He then attended Cornell University, where he received an M.S. in physics. Brendan will receive his medical degree from Ohio State University in 2002. He will begin his residency in neurology at the Cleveland Clinic in July of 2002.

Helen J. Kim
Class of 2003
Medical College of Virginia/Virginia Commonwealth University, Richmond,
 Virginia

Helen was born and raised in Los Angeles, CA. She attended UCLA for undergraduate study, where she majored in microbiology and molecular genetics and received a specialization in Asian-American Studies. She remained at UCLA to receive a master's in public health with a focus on epidemiology. She will receive her medical degree in 2003 from the Medical College of Virginia/Virginia Commonwealth University. Whenever she finds free time, Helen enjoys surfing and snowboarding.

Shane C. Kim
Class of 2002
University of Kansas School Of Medicine
Kansas City, Kansas

Shane received his medical degree in 2002 from the University of Kansas School of Medicine in Kansas City, Kansas. He did his undergraduate work at the University of Kansas in Lawrence, Kansas, majoring in microbiology. He is currently pursuing a residency in general surgery at the University of Kansas Medical Center. His original hometown is Topeka, Kansas.

Jennifer W. Jung
Class of 2003
Jefferson Medical College, Philadelphia, Pennsylvania

Jennifer is currently a third-year medical student at Jefferson Medical College in Philadelphia, PA. She received her undergraduate degree in classics: Latin from Brown University in Providence, RI.

Danny Liaw
Class of 2002
Columbia University College of Physicians and Surgeons
New York, New York

Born in Taichung, Taiwan, Danny grew up in the suburbs of Philadelphia. He majored in molecular biology and biochemistry at Wesleyan University in Connecticut and afterwards spent two years as a research technician at Thomas Jefferson University. He then entered Columbia University's M.D./Ph.D. program where he did his doctorate on the identification and characterization of a tumor suppressor gene. He will be doing a residency in internal medicine at Beth Israel Deaconess Medical Center in Boston.

Heather Malm
Class of 2002
Des Moines University–Osteopathic Medical Center
Des Moines, Iowa

Heather was born in Boulder, Colorado, and grew up in the small town of Louisville, Colorado. She completed her undergraduate studies at the University of San Francisco, where she received her degree in biology. Heather received her medical degree in 2002 from Des Moines University in Iowa. She will complete her residency in emergency medicine at the York Hospital/Pennsylvania State University program in York, Pennsylvania.

Edward C. Miner
Class 2002
Washington University, Saint Louis, Missouri

Ed grew up in Springville, Utah, and earned a degree in molecular biology from Brigham Young University. He received an academic scholarship to attend Washington University School of Medicine, graduating in 2002. He is currently a resident in internal medicine at the Mayo Clinic.

John Nguyen

Class of 2003
University of Texas Medical Branch, Galveston, Texas

Born in Vietnam, John grew up in Saigon before moving with his family to Houston, Texas, at the age of thirteen. He graduated summa cum laude from the University of Houston with a bachelor of science in biology. John is currently attending the University of Texas Medical Branch at Galveston and is expected to earn his medical degree in 2003.

Nancy Pandhi

Family Practice Resident
Shenandoah Family Practice Residency
Front Royal, Virginia

Nancy received her medical degree in 2001 from the Virginia Commonwealth University. She attended the University of Chicago for undergraduate study, where she was a political science major. Her hobbies are gardening, reading, and hiking—and she plans to add a new one each year of residency.

Avi Patel

Class of 2003
New York University, New York, New York

Avi was born in Queens, New York, and raised in the town of Edison, New Jersey. He attended college at Johns Hopkins University, majoring in biology and minoring in science, medicine, and culture. Following college, Avi took a year off from school to work in health policy in Washington, D.C., and travel. He is currently enrolled in NYU School of Medicine, from which he will graduate in 2003 with a medical degree.

Diane Rychlik

Class of 2002
Spartan Health Sciences University School of Medicine
  Vieux Fort, St. Lucia

Born in Chicago, IL, Diane has always enjoyed working with people. She completed a B.A. in philosophy at the University of Illinois at Chicago. From there, Diane decided to do something different by applying to a foreign medical school from which she will be graduating and starting a family practice residency.

Alex Sassani, CPA

Class of 2002
University of California, San Diego
La Jolla, California

Alex attended the University of Southern California as an undergraduate. After working for Ernst & Young, LLP for several years, he changed careers and entered medical school. Alex plans on a career in academic medicine and administration. He has published several articles and has teaching experience both at USC and commercial test preparation companies.

Christopher Todd Starnes
Class of 2002
University of Virginia
Charlottesville, Virginia

Chris received his doctor of medicine degree in 2002 from the University of Virginia, in Charlottesville, VA. He grew up in the coal town of Wise, VA, where he also attended college at Clinch Valley. While at Clinch Valley he met his wife, Katie Starnes, who is a medical student at Eastern Virginia Medical School. Chris entered residency training in internal medicine at the University of South Carolina in July 2002 with high aspirations of teaching and pursuing fellowship training.

Joshua D. Valtos, MD
Class of 2002
Emory University School of Medicine
Atlanta, Georgia

Josh was born and raised in Shiloh, Illinois. He attended Southern Illinois University at Carbondale where he earned degrees in zoology and physiology and met his wife, Amanda. He graduated from Emory University School of Medicine. Josh is currently a resident in family medicine at the University of Missouri-Columbia.

REVIEWERS

Jill Albrecht
Class of 2003
SUNY at Buffalo
Buffalo, New York

Alexander Ayzengart
Class of 2003
University of Michigan Medical School
Ann Arbor, Michigan

Nikil Bhagat
Class of 2003
UMDNJ-NJMS
Newark, New Jersy

Kelly Bromfield
Class of 2003
University of Michigan Medical School
Ann Arbor, Michigan

Hon Cheung Chan
Class of 2003
SUNY Stonybrook School of Medicine
Stonybrook, New York

Patrick Chen
Class of 2003
University of Michigan Medical School
Ann Arbor, Michigan

Mabelle Cohen
Class of 2003
Finch University of Health Sciences/Chicago Medical
  School
Chicago, Illinois

Michele Irons
Class of 2003
MCP-Hahnemann
Philadelphia, Pennsylvania

Faizi Asim Jamal
Class of 2003
University of California at Irvine College of Medicine
Irvine, California

Jennifer Jung
Class of 2003
Jefferson Medical College: Thomas Jefferson University
  Philadelphia, Pennsylvania

Chad Kliger
Class of 2003
Temple University School of Medicine
Philadelphia, Pennsylvania

Lisa Knust
Class of 2003
Medical College of Virginia of Virginia Commonwealth
  University
Richmond, Virginia

Juliette Lee
Class of 2003
Columbia University School of Medicine
New York, New York

Janos Marozsan
Class of 2004
St. Matthew's University School of Medicine
Oviedo, Florida

Innocent Monya-Tambi
Class of 2003
Howard University College of Medicine
Washington, DC

Jill Moore
Class of 2003
University of Utah School of Medicine
Salt Lake City, Utah

Karen Moore
Class of 2003
Duke University School of Medicine
Durham, North Carolina

Nkiruka Ohameje
Class of 2003
MCP Hahnemann School of Medicine
Philadelphia, Pennsylvania

Julie Phillips
Class of 2003
University of Michigan Medical School
Ann Arbor, Michigan

Corinne LeVon Quinn
Class of 2003
MCP Hahnemann School of Medicine
Philadelphia, Pennsylvania

Christian Ramers
Class of 2003
University of California, Los Angeles College of Medicine
Los Angeles, California

Victor R. Rodriguez
Class of 2003
Tufts University School of Medicine
Boston, Massachusetts

Brook Rosman
Class of 2003
MCP Hahnemann School of Medicine
Philadelphia, Pennsylvania

Ruth Sanchez
Class of 2003
UMDNJ-NJMS
Newark, New Jersey

Christopher Scott
Class of 2003
Brody School of Medicine
Greenville, North Carolina

Amish C. Shah
Class of 2003
University of Alabama at Birmingham
Birmingham, Alabama

Shawn M. Smith
Class of 2003
University of Utah School of Medicine
Salt Lake City, Utah

Can Tang
Class of 2003
University of Arizona College of Medicine
Tucson, Arizona

Floyd Thompson, III
Class of 2003
University of Arizona College of Medicine
Tucson, Arizona

Jason Tinley
Class of 2003
Medical College of Georgia
Augusta, Georgia

Alexander C. Tsai
Class of 2003
Case Western Reserve University School of Medicine
Cleveland, Ohio

Henry K. Tsai
Class of 2002
Harvard Medical School
Boston, Massachusetts

Henry Tsay
Class of 2003
Temple University School of Medicine
Philadelphia, Pennsylvania

Amber M. Tyler
Class of 2003
University of Nebraska
Omaha, Nebraska

Lisa Usdan
Class of 2003
University of Tennessee College of Medicine
Memphis, Tennessee

Nilong Vyas
Class of 2004
Louisiana State University Health Sciences Center
New Orleans, Louisiana

NORMAL LABORATORY VALUES

Hematology

White Blood Cell Count (total leukocytes)	4500–11,000/mm^3

Leukocytes, Differential

Polymorphonuclear leukocytes (PMN) (segmented neutrophils)	54–62%
Banded neutrophils	3–5%
Myelocytes	0%
Lymphocytes	25–33%
Monocytes	3–7%
Eosinophoils	1–3%
Basophils	0–1%
Platelets	150,000–400,000/mm^3
Reticulocytes	0.5–1.5% of erythrocytes

Hematocrit

Males	40–54 mL/dL
Females	37–47 mL/dL
Newborns	49–54 mL/dL
Children (varies with age)	35–49 mL/dL

Hemoglobin

Males	13–18 g/dL
Females	12–16 g/dL
Newborns	16.5–19.5 g/dL
Children (varies with age)	11.2–16.5 g/dL

Erythrocyte Sedimentation Rate

Wintrobe

Male	0–5 mm/h
Female	0–15 mm/h

Westergren

Male	0–15 mm/h
Female	0–20 mm/h

Red Cell Indices

Mean corpuscular hemoglobin (MCH)	26–34 pg/cell
Mean corpuscular volume (MCV)	80–96 um^3
Mean corpuscular hemoglobin concentration	32–36 gm/dL

Coagulation

Prothrombin time (PT)	12.0–14.0 seconds
Partial thromboplastin time (PTT)	20–35 seconds

Serum Electrolytes

Sodium	135–145 mEq/L
Potassium	3.5–5.0 mEq/L
Chloride	96–106 mEq/L
Carbon dioxide	24–31 mEq/L
Bicarbonate (venous)	23–29 mEq/L
Bicarbonate (arterial)	21–27 mEq/L

Blood Gases (Arterial)

PaO$_2$	80–100 mmHg
SaO$_2$	95–98%
PCO$_2$	35–45 mmHg

Blood Lipids (Serum)

Total cholesterol	<200 mg/dL
LDL cholesterol	60–180 mg/dL
HDL cholesterol	30–80 mg/dL
Triglycerides	40–150 mg/dL

Cerebrospinal Fluid

Glucose	40–70 mg/dL
Protein	12–60 mg/dL
Colorless	
Clear	
White blood cells	0–30/mm^3
Red blood cells	0

Miscellaneous Chemistries

Serum Bilirubin (Adult)

Conjugated	0.1–0.4 mg/dL
Total	0.3–1.1 mg/dL
Glucose (fasting)	70–115 mg/dL
BUN	11–23 mg/dL
Creatinine	0.6–1.2 mg/dL

Thyroid

TSH	0.4–4.8 uIU/ml
Free thyroxine (FT$_4$)	0.9–2.1 ng/dL
Thyroxine (T$_4$)	4.5–12.0 ug/dL
Triiodothyronine (T$_3$)	70–190 ng/dL

Prostate

Prostate Specific Antigen (PSA) ng of PSA/L

Age	Whites	Blacks
40–49	0.0–2.5	0.0–2.0
50–59	0.0–3.5	0.0–4.0
60–69	0.0–3.5	0.0–4.5
70–79	0.0–3.5	0.0–5.5

CONTENT INDEX

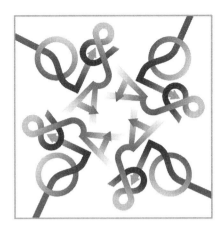

QUESTIONS
BLOCK 1

1. A 75-year-old male with a 100-pack-per-year history of smoking and known lung cancer presents to his doctor with hoarseness. He has no other complaints. CT reveals a left apical lung mass with no involvement of the vocal cords. However, exam reveals paralysis of the left vocal cord. You suspect that a nerve has been damaged. Which of the following is true regarding that nerve?

   A. It is not a branch of CN X.
   B. On the left side, it can be found wrapped around the arch of the aorta.
   C. Cranial nerves C3-C5 contribute to this nerve.
   D. It is responsible for autonomic innervation up to the splenic flexure.
   E. It is responsible for taste in the posterior portion of the tongue.

2. A 42-year-old woman, in the process of a divorce, comes to your office for therapy. She describes her recent participation in and satisfaction from playing in a hockey league, whereas previously she did not engage in such physically aggressive activities. Which of the following defense mechanisms best characterizes her behavior?

   A. Sublimation
   B. Rationalization
   C. Altruism
   D. Suppression
   E. Projection

3. A 52-year-old homeless man presents to your emergency room after having been found on the street having a seizure. As he is being wheeled in, the paramedics report a pulse of 110, BP 165/100,

RR 28, T 101.5°F. You note that the patient is continuing to convulse and is profusely diaphoretic. You control the seizures by placing him on chlordiazepoxide. Further examination demonstrates crackles in both lower lung fields and pitting edema of the lower extremities. The chest x-ray demonstrates an enlarged heart. You continue to treat him as indicated for his immediate and chronic conditions. Three hours later you repeat a neurological exam and discover mild nystagmus, ophthalmoplegia, and wrist drop. Of the multiple problems this man faces due to his condition, you must recognize and immediately begin treatment for the possible deficiency of a certain enzymatic cofactor. Which of the following biochemical pathways contains an enzyme that requires this cofactor?

   A. Glycolysis
   B. Hexose monophosphate shunt
   C. Malate shuttle
   D. Gluconeogenesis
   E. Fatty acid beta-oxidation

4. A 6-month-old child presents to the clinic with an explosive cough and a 10-day history of choking spells and worsening cough. When asked about immunizations given to the child, none had been given because of religious objections. A CBC showed lymphocytosis. What causative agent should be suspected?

   A. Respiratory syncytial virus
   B. *Bordetella pertussis*
   C. *Haemophilus influenzae*
   D. *Streptococcus pneumoniae*
   E. *Legionella pneumophila*

5. A 22-year-old male college student presents to the ER with recent onset of painful joints, eye pain, and dysuria. He is sexually active with multiple women and never uses condoms. His past medical history is positive for psoriasis and multiple sexually transmitted diseases. He denies any recent GI upset. He has a brother with ankylosing spondylitis. A KUB reveals no inflammation of the sacroiliac joints. The most likely disease process is:

   A. Reiter's syndrome
   B. Psoriatic arthropathy
   C. Reactive arthropathy
   D. Rheumatoid arthritis
   E. Ankylosing spondylitis

6. A 35-year-old white female patient presents with a history of morning stiffness, fatigue, and joint swelling and tenderness of several months' duration. On examination she has symmetrical, swollen, and painful joints. Lab reports show elevated blood levels of creatinine and BUN. What drug should be used to bring her arthritis under control?

A. Celecoxib

B. Methotrexate

C. Indomethacin

D. Acetaminophen

E. Cyclosporine

7. A 65-year-old man with a history of alcoholism presents to your clinic with multiple complaints, including severe hemorrhoids. In addition, he was hospitalized several months ago for bleeding gastric varices, which were ligated. On physical examination, you palpate an enlarged spleen, observe a dilated venous plexus around his umbilicus, and confirm the presence of hemorrhoids. He does not have lower extremity edema and denies shortness of breath, chest pain, or history of heart trouble. His history and physical findings indicate which of the following physiological abnormalities?

A. Increased portal venous pressure

B. Increased central arterial pressure

C. Increased central venous pressure

D. Increased pulmonary arterial pressure

8. A 75-year-old male presents to his primary care doctor complaining of right scalp and head pain of an increasingly severe nature. The symptoms began as fever, fatigue, and weight loss; the head and scalp pain developed after several months. On physical examination there is tenderness to touch in the right temporal area. Which of the following is most likely true regarding his condition?

A. Vision is rarely affected.

B. Coronary arteries are frequently affected.

C. It is frequently associated with cerebrovascular accidents.

D. Granulomatous inflammation of the affected arteries is usually seen.

E. Most patients with temporal arteritis are males less than 50 years old.

9. A 45-year-old white male presented with epigastric pain of several weeks' duration. He was diagnosed with a duodenal ulcer. **See Figure 9.** He was given a combination therapy of bismuth subsalicylate, metronidazole, and tetracycline. The most likely causative agent is:

A. *Entamoeba histolytica*

B. *Escherichia coli*

C. *Helicobacter pylori*

D. *Salmonella typhi*

E. *Campylobacter jejuni*

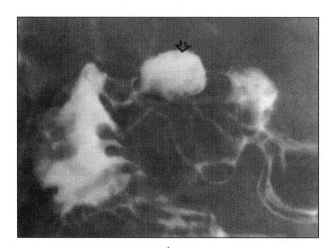

A

B

Figure 9 Reproduced with permission from Armstrong. Diagnostic Imaging, 4/e. Blackwell Science, Ltd., 1998.

10. A 76-year-old woman presents to your office for an initial visit. Her blood pressure is found to be 180/100 mm Hg, and renal bruits are heard on auscultation of the abdomen. Renal angiogram shows severe bilateral renal artery stenosis. While making arrangements for angioplasty and stenting of her renal arteries, which of the following blood pressure medications is contraindicated in this patient?

A. Hydralazine
B. Metoprolol
C. Amlodipine
D. Captopril

11. A 39-year-old man sustains a gunshot wound to the right shoulder. On examination, he has difficulty with right arm abduction more than 45° and loses sensation on the lateral side of the right shoulder. Radiographic images suggest a fracture at the surgical neck of the humerus. **See Figure 11.** What artery could be damaged in this injury?

A. Circumflex humeral artery
B. Subscapular artery
C. Thoracoacromial artery
D. Brachial artery
E. Axillary artery

12. A female infant began experiencing postfeeding vomiting and diarrhea seven days after birth. By six months of age, the baby presented with failure to thrive, was visibly jaundiced, had increased urinary excretion of albumen and sugar, and was found on exam to have hepatomegaly as well as cataracts. Family history was positive for a high frequency of neonatal death secondary to bacterial infection. The patient most likely has a defect in which metabolic enzyme?

A. Aldolase B
B. Lactase
C. Galactose 1-phosphate uridyl transferase
D. Fructokinase
E. Glucose-6-phosphate dehydrogenase

13. A 6-year-old boy presents to the clinic with a history and EEG findings suggestive of grand mal epilepsy. You elect to place him on phenytoin. Which of the following best characterizes this drug?

A. Mechanism of action is blockade of Na+ channels
B. Treatment of choice for absence seizures
C. Inhibits p450 system
D. Chronic use can result in gingival hypoplasia in children
E. No known teratogenicity

14. Which of the following is true regarding stages of sleep?

A. Approximately 75% of sleep is spent in REM sleep.
B. EEG waveform pattern during the awake and alert state (beta) is the same pattern that is seen during REM sleep.
C. Acetylcholine is the key neurotransmitter in initiating sleep.
D. Dreaming occurs during stage 1, or lighter sleep.
E. Imipramine increases the length of time spent in stage 4, the deepest non-REM sleep.

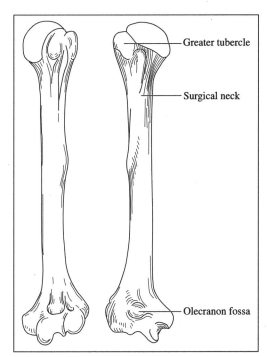

— Greater tubercle

— Surgical neck

— Olecranon fossa

Figure 11

15. A 58-year-old male with a long history of chronic obstructive pulmonary disease (COPD) comes to his private medical doctor complaining of a cold and the onset of shortness of breath. The patient has always been a heavy smoker of 4 to 5 packs per day with a chronic productive cough that has gotten worse over the past two nights. The patient is an obese man, appears mildly cyanotic, and labors to breathe with his expiration prolonged. The values on the oxygen-hemoglobin dissociation curve that best reflect this patient's condition are:

	PaO$_2$ (mmHg)	% Saturation of Hemoglobin
A.	90	95
B.	80	90
C.	70	60
D.	60	90
E.	50	85

16. A 24-year-old female presented with abdominal pain and a pelvic mass that had developed over a short period of time. She had surgery to remove a tumor that was found to involve a single ovary. Histology revealed characteristic glomerulus-like structures of germ cells surrounding germ cells enveloping a central blood vessel (Schiller-Duval bodies) with conspicuous intracellular and extracellular hyaline droplets that can be stained for:

A. B-hCG

B. AFP

C. Estrogen

D. Androgen

E. Thyroid hormone

17. A 12-year-old boy is brought to the emergency room with difficulty breathing. On exam, he has expiratory wheezes over all lung fields and demonstrates retractions on inspection. He is unable to speak in complete sentences. Of the medicine he might have, the one that would have on its label "for prevention only" would be:

A. Ipratropium

B. Albuterol

C. Magnesium sulfate

D. Prednisone

E. Cromolyn sodium

18. A 3-year-old child in a third-world country subsists on a diet exclusively of taro root and some fruits. Physical examination reveals a lethargic child with hepatomegaly and a distended abdomen. Which of the following is most likely responsible for this child's appearance?

A. Inadequate vitamin C consumption

B. Inadequate vitamin D consumption

C. Inadequate consumption of protein

D. Inadequate consumption of fat

19. A 22-year-old male presents to your clinic with difficulty moving his right arm. Two days ago he was playing tackle football with his college roommates, when he got a "stinger" after a hard hit that flexed his neck laterally to the left. He didn't think much about it but hasn't been able to use the arm since the event. You order nerve studies to determine the site of the lesion. The report shows an upper-trunk lesion. Which action do you expect to be normal on exam?

A. External rotation of arm

B. Abduction of arm at shoulder

C. Sensory deficit on the lateral side of the distal arm

D. Extension of forearm at the elbow

E. Weakness in flexion of the arm at the shoulder

20. A 23-year-old white female comes to your office with a complaint of having difficulty with interpersonal relationships with her coworkers and supervisor. She seems to have little insight into what her problem may be. Which of the following is an OBJECTIVE psychological test that you may wish to administer?

A. Thematic Apperception Test (TAT)

B. Rorschach Ink Blot

C. Minnesota Multiphasic Personality Inventory (MMPI)

D. Draw a Person Test

E. Sentence Completion Test (SCT)

21. A 22-year-old woman comes to your office after returning from college spring break in Florida. In the last two days she has had pain and frequency when she urinates. She has had a slight fever, but no other symptoms. She is on no medications, has no allergies, and no other medical conditions except requiring eyeglasses for reading. After getting a urine sample, the culture comes back as "Many gram-positive cocci which are catalase positive but coagulase negative." The most likely organism is:

A. *Staph aureus*
B. *Staph saprophyticus*
C. *Strep faecalis*
D. *E. coli*
E. *Neisseria gonorrhoeae*

22. A 63-year-old white woman comes to your office as a new patient. She complains of weakness and a tremor. On examination she has a masklike facies and exhibits pill rolling with her fingers and muscle rigidity. Which of the following drugs would exacerbate her Parkinson's disease?

A. Amantadine
B. Bromocriptine
C. Chlorpromazine
D. Levodopa/Carbidopa
E. Pergolide
F. Selegiline
G. Tolcapone
H. Trihexyphenidyl

23. A 35-year-old woman reports an occasional burning sensation in the center of her chest that is partially relieved by antacids. She desires medication to more completely reduce her symptoms. Medications that act at which of the following sites will **more completely** reduce gastric acid secretion?

A. Histamine (H_2) receptor
B. H^+, K^+-ATPase
C. Acetylcholine receptor
D. Gastrin receptor

24. A 45-year-old white female presents to your office with several complaints. She is having trouble sleeping and feels that her life is dull and that she is unappreciated by her husband and family. Her job, in her words, is "dead-end and boring." She has a poor appetite and appears angry. What disorder is she most likely to have?

A. Bipolar disorder
B. Autism
C. Major depressive disorder
D. Schizophrenia
E. Attention deficit disorder

25. A 30-year-old black, obese woman is seen for a six-month history of joint pain and fatigue. She complains of several episodes of skin rashes over her face and neck, especially when working outdoors. Her fatigue prevents her from going out anymore. It is discovered that the patient has renal insufficiency. The laboratory results are also positive for antidouble stranded DNA antibodies as well as for elevated serum levels of ANA. The patient is started on prednisolone, shows clinical improvement, and is discharged to home. The patient returns two weeks later with oral ulcers, increased weight gain, a fasting blood glucose level of 200, hypertension of 160/100, and a moonlike face that is round and plethoric. What is the most appropriate next step?

A. Perform a dexamethasone suppression test.
B. Give a subcutaneous injection of insulin.
C. Order a 24-hour urinary free cortisol determination.
D. Taper prednisolone to the lowest therapeutic dose.
E. Request a CT-scan of the pituitary gland.

26. A 60-year-old man with a 90-pack-per-year history of cigarette smoking presented with productive cough, 20-pound weight loss over the past year, and dyspnea. A complete work-up revealed a 3-cm mass in the right upper lung lobe. **See Figure 26.** For which of the following would it be inappropriate to treat with surgical resection?

A. Squamous cell carcinoma
B. Adenocarcinoma
C. Small-cell carcinoma
D. Large-cell carcinoma
E. Hamartoma

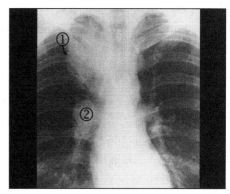

Figure 26 Reproduced with permission from Armstrong. Diagnostic Imaging, 4/e. Blackwell Science, Ltd., 1998.

27. A medical student sticks himself with a needle while drawing blood from a patient in the emergency room. He has received a complete series of hepatitis B immunizations and has confirmed the presence of anti-HBs antibodies. Which of the following types of hepatitis is this student most at risk for?

    A. Hepatitis A
    B. Hepatitis B
    C. Hepatitis C
    D. Hepatitis D
    E. Hepatitis E

28. A 26-year-old woman comes into the asthma clinic with complaints of increased asthma attacks. She had been prescribed an albuterol inhaler to use when she suffers an attack. For several years, she only had two to three attacks per month, each time relieved by her inhaler. However, in the last two weeks, she has been experiencing three to four attacks per week. She denies any other allergic symptoms, change in work, or new pets. What should be done to manage this patient's asthma?

    A. Continue the albuterol inhaler.
    B. Discontinue albuterol and begin inhaled fluticasone.
    C. Add inhaled fluticasone to the albuterol.
    D. Add ipratropium bromide to the albuterol.
    E. Add a leukotriene inhibitor.

29. A 56-year-old man with hypercholesterolemia, diabetes, and a 60-pack-per-year history of smoking arrives in the ER. Unfortunately, all the interns, residents, and nurses are stuck at home due to a major snowstorm. The patient tells you that after shoveling the driveway this morning he felt like an elephant sat on his chest. His wife stated that he also looked sweaty and short of breath. **See Figure 29.** After looking at the EKG, you notice Q waves in the anterior leads V1-V6 with ST segment depression. While still standing over the EKG, the cardiology fellow asks you which artery you are most concerned about. You answer:

    A. Right main coronary artery (RCA)
    B. Circumflex branch of the left coronary artery
    C. Left anterior descending coronary artery (LAD)
    D. Posterior descending artery (PDA)
    E. Thoracoacromial artery

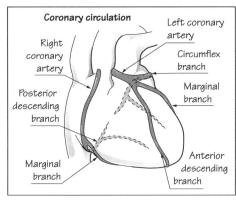

Figure 29 Reproduced with permission from Aaronson. The Cardiovascular System at a Glance. Blackwell Science, Ltd., 1999.

30. An infant is born at term and maintains a slight degree of cyanosis for the first 24 hours of life, which then spontaneously clears. Chest x-ray was normal. Which of the following statements about oxygen bound by hemoglobin is correct?

    A. Carbon dioxide increases the affinity of oxygen to hemoglobin by binding to the amino groups of the chains.
    B. The oxygen affinity for adult hemoglobin is greater than for neonates.
    C. The hemoglobin dimer binds two molecules of 2,3 BPG.
    D. The greater saturation of hemoglobin corresponds to the greater affinity for oxygen.
    E. The increase in pH values decreases hemoglobin's affinity for oxygen.

31. A 33-year-old woman has a progressively enlarging midline neck mass. She has heat intolerance, increased sweating, weight loss, tachycardia, fatigue, and weakness. **See Figure 31.** Laboratory results show increased T3 and T4 levels. What is the most likely etiology of her symptoms?

    A. Increased thyroid peroxidase
    B. Increased thyroid deiodinase
    C. Increased thyroglobulin
    D. Increased thyroid stimulating immunoglobulin
    E. None of the above

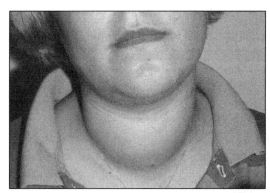

Figure 31 Reproduced with permission from Clement. Blueprints Q&A Step 2. Blackwell Science, Inc., 2001.

32. A 53-year-old man comes to the primary-care clinic for a follow-up appointment. On his previous visit, you drew blood and sent it for a lipid profile. See **Table 32** for the results.

The patient does not smoke or drink and has no family history of heart disease or stroke. His blood pressure is 124/82 mm Hg. Which of the following antihyperlipidemic agents best suits this patient?

A. Simvastatin

B. Niacin

C. Gemfibrozil

D. Cholestyramine

E. None of the above

Table 32

LIPID PROFILE	
Total cholesterol	215 mg/dL
HDL	33 mg/dL
LDL	119 mg/dL
Triglycerides	313 mg/dL

33. The gram-positive bacteria *Bacillus anthracis* is used in biological warfare applications due to its spore-forming ability and to the potential lethality of human disease caused by inhalation of these spores. Which of the following contributes to the virulence of *B. anthracis*?

A. Polypeptide capsule

B. Edema factor

C. Shiga-like toxin

D. Lethal factor

E. A, B, and D

34. A 39-year-old married woman comes into your office for a routine physical examination. In the waiting room she is fixing her hair in a mirror. She is dressed in bright colors and a fur coat, is wearing excessive makeup and perfume, alternates between crying and laughing, and is inappropriately flirtatious during the interview. Her presentation is most consistent with which of the following personality disorders?

A. Borderline

B. Narcissistic

C. Dependent

D. Paranoid

E. Histrionic

35. A 15-year-old girl presents to the pediatrician with ankle pain and fever. Her symptoms began two days ago, and she had a sore throat three weeks ago. On cardiac auscultation, there is a II/VI systolic murmur. The physician recommends that she have an echocardiogram of the heart done. Which of the following statements concerning AV valves are correct?

I. Papillary muscles facilitate opening of the AV valves.
II. Prolapse of the mitral valve can cause severe pulmonary edema.
III. The AV valve in the right ventricle is called the bicuspid valve.
IV. *Staphylococcus aureus* is the most common cause of mitral valve damage.
V. Mitral valve prolapse occurs during systole.

A. I, II, III

B. II, III, IV

C. III, IV, V

D. I, II, V

E. I, II, III, IV

36. A 45-year-old white businessman who frequently travels overseas has a gradual onset of arthralgia, arthritis, fatigue, and headache for several months. He also has episodes of diarrhea and steatorrhea. Physical exam shows lymphadenopathy and skin hyperpigmentation. Laboratory results, including stool culture, are negative. The patient's symptoms subsided after empirical treatment with antibiotics. What would you find in an intestinal mucosa biopsy of this patient?

A. Fibrinopurulent-necrotic debris and mucus adhesion

B. Marked atrophy of villi

C. Variable villus blunting

D. Crypt abscesses and lesions extending to muscularis propria

E. Distended macrophages containing PAS positive granules and *Tropheryma whippelii*

37. Mr. Gomez, one of your patients, returns to your office two weeks after you have prescribed captopril. He is complaining of a new symptom that you immediately recognize as a side effect of this medication. This symptom is most likely:

A. Increased energy

B. Decreased sex drive

C. Increased volume and frequency of urination

D. New-onset cough

E. New-onset decreased night vision

38. Which of the following statements about viruses is true?

A. Viruses must be infectious in order to survive in nature.

B. Viruses are living organisms.

C. A viral genome may be RNA or DNA, but not both.

D. Some viruses are surrounded by a membrane composed of glycoproteins, proteins, and lipids.

E. All of the above

F. A, C, and D

39. A 78-year-old man comes to a psychiatrist having been referred by his family physician. He has recently lost his wife and has been experiencing anhedonia, anorexia, and insomnia. He has no other medical problems; his biggest concern is his inability to sleep through the night. Based on this information, in addition to counseling you decide to prescribe:

A. Amitriptyline

B. Olanzapine

C. Paroxetine

D. Tranylcypromine

E. Electroshock therapy

40. A 45-year-old man is concerned about increasing breast size bilaterally. He does not take any steroids and is not a chronic alcoholic. He suffers from epigastric pain and hypertension. Which of the following most likely has caused his gynecomastia?

A. Cimetidine

B. Phenytoin

C. Carbamazepine

D. Felodipine

E. Quinidine

41. A 35-year-old white female presents to your office for the first time. She has a staring gaze with wide and protuberant eyes. Her history reveals that she is usually anxious and sometimes has heart palpitations. **See Figure 41.** Which of the following is most likely correct?

A. Her TSH is above 5.0.

B. She suffers from thyroid carcinoma.

C. She suffers from thyroid adenoma.

D. She suffers from Hashimoto's thyroiditis.

E. None of the above

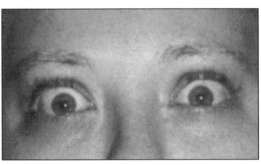

Figure 41   Reproduced with permission from Clement. Blueprints Q&A Step 2. Blackwell Science, Inc., 2001.

42. An 18-year-old college student comes in to the student health service complaining of severe headache and photophobia. She tells you the headache has been present for one day and getting worse. On examination, there is meningismus and you notice red spots on her thighs that do not blanch when they are pressed. A lumbar puncture is done with the following results:

Pressure: 200 mm CSF
WBC count: 3500 cells/mm³ with 85% PMNs
Glucose: 28 mg/dL
Protein: 113 mg/dL

What organism is the most likely cause of this patient's illness?

A. *Streptococcus pneumoniae*

B. *Staphylococcus aureus*

C. *Listeria monocytogenes*

D. *Neisseria meningitidis*

E. *Streptococcus agalactiae*

43. A 16-year-old female, belonging to an upper-middle-class family, presents to her primary care physician's office for her annual sports physical for the high school track team. Her weight is 110 pounds, which is 10 pounds below her ideal body weight. Her physical exam is otherwise normal. The patient states she has been feeling fine and doing well in school, but she admits to not having her menstrual period for the past three months. Her mother relates that her daughter exercises excessively and she has witnessed her daughter purging after a large meal on a few occasions. This patient does not meet the criteria for the diagnosis of anorexia nervosa because:

A. She binges and purges.

B. She has amenorrhea.

C. She belongs to a high socioeconomic class.

D. Her weight does not meet the diagnostic criteria.

E. She is female.

44. A 48-year-old male presents for a physical exam. His general exam is within normal limits except that he is somewhat overweight. Laboratory testing reveals that his total cholesterol is 250 mg/dL. You give him a one-month trial of cholesterol-lowering drug A, at a dose of 200 mg/day. At the end of the month his cholesterol is 200 mg/dL. The next month you stop drug A and give him drug B at a dose of 100 mg/day. His cholesterol at the end of the month taking drug B is 200 mg/dL. You could infer that these two drugs have the same:

A. Potency

B. Efficacy

C. ED (effective dose)

D. LD_{50}

E. None of the above

45. A 22-year-old female complains of a discharge from her vagina and pelvic pain. She has no itching but is worried because of the discharge. She is sexually active. Pelvic exam reveals a mucopurulent discharge with a positive Chandelier sign. Cultures show a gram-negative, nonencapsulated, oxidase-positive diplococci that does not ferment maltose. You also run a second test, fluorescent antibody stain, looking for any cytoplasmic inclusions, for which results are pending. You begin treating her with ceftriaxone and azithromycin since you suspect:

A. Genital herpes

B. Candidiasis

C. Gonorrhea/chlamydia

D. *Trichomonas vaginalis*

E. *Gardnerella vaginalis*

46. Which of the following genetic defects in the α-globin gene leads to a mild microcytic anemia without hemolysis and no dependence on transfusion? **See Table 46.**

Positions A1 and A2 represent the two alleles of the α-globin gene on one chromosome and B1 and B2 represent the two alleles of the α-globin gene on the other chromosome. α represents that a copy of the allele is present and a dash means it is absent.

Table 46

	A1	A2	B1	B2
A.	α	α	α	α
B.	α	α	α	—
C.	α	α	—	—
D.	α	—	—	—
E.	—	—	—	—

47. A patient presents to your office stating that he woke up in the middle of the night with extreme pain of his big toe metatarsal joint. It is red, warm, swollen, and extremely tender. You start him on colchicine. The mechanism of action of this drug is to:

A. Disrupt the mobility of granulocytes and inhibit the synthesis and release of leukotrienes

B. Reduce the production of uric acid by inhibiting the last two steps in uric acid biosynthesis

C. Block the proximal tubular resorption of uric acid

D. Irreversibly acetylate cyclooxygenase

E. Disrupt the cell wall of the bacteria causing the inflammation

48. A 9-year-old boy with a long history of pulmonary problems is admitted to your pediatrics team. The patient coughs up copious amounts of green sputum while examining him. His past medical history is significant for meconium ileus as a newborn and chronic sinusitis. In addition, he typically has foul-smelling, oily stools.

Vitals: Temperature 38.5°C   Pulse 70

BP 110/65   Respiratory rate 30

Oxygen Saturation 90% on room air

Which of the following statements is true?

A. A sweat test shows decreased chloride concentration.

B. He will have elevated pancreatic amylase levels.

C. Patients with this disease show hypoinflation on a chest x-ray.

D. His pulmonary function tests will show hypoxemia and an increase in FVC (forced vital capacity).

E. The disease is caused by a mutation in the CFTR gene.

49. In a small town in the United States with a total population of 3000 (1600 men and 1400 women), 50 individuals were newly diagnosed with a chronic but nonfatal disease between January 1, 2001, and December 31, 2001. Up until January 1, 2001, a total of 100 people had already been diagnosed with the same disease. Assuming that no one in this population has died in the past five years, and no one has moved into or out of this town, what is the prevalence ratio of this disease in 2001 among this town's population?

A. 50/1600

B. 150/3000

C. 50/3000

D. 150/1400

E. 50/1400

50. An elderly man is undergoing open prostatectomy. During the operation he was transfused with four units of packed RBCs. Soon after the operation, his catheter becomes dark, his hematocrit drops, and he is hypotensive. What is the most appropriate management at this time?

A. Transfuse more RBCs

B. Epinephrine

C. Heparin IV

D. Vitamin K

E. Fresh frozen plasma

BLOCK I - ANSWER KEY

1-B	14-B	27-C	39-C
2-A	15-C	28-C	40-A
3-B	16-B	29-C	41-E
4-B	17-E	30-D	42-D
5-A	18-C	31-D	43-D
6-B	19-D	32-C	44-B
7-A	20-C	33-E	45-C
8-D	21-B	34-E	46-C
9-C	22-C	35-D	47-A
10-D	23-B	36-E	48-E
11-A	24-C	37-D	49-B
12-C	25-D	38-E	50-E
13-A	26-C		

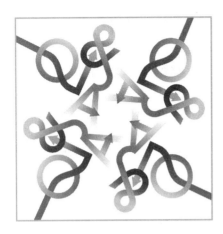

ANSWERS
BLOCK 1

1. B The nerve described in this question is the recurrent laryngeal nerve. On the left side, this nerve wraps around the arch of the aorta.

A. The recurrent laryngeal nerve is a branch of CN X.

C. It is a branch of CN X.

D. This describes the vagus nerve, of which the recurrent laryngeal is a branch but is not true for the recurrent laryngeal.

E. The recurrent laryngeal nerve has no special sense functions.

2. A Ego defenses are unconscious reactions to psychological stresses and are categorized into mature and less mature defenses. Sublimation, a mature ego defense, is the transformation of unacceptable wishes or urges into socially acceptable actions. Examples include using anger or aggression to succeed in sports or business.

B. Rationalization is a less mature defense in which irrational thoughts are made to seem reasonable.

C. Altruism, a mature ego defense, is unselfishly helping others.

D. Suppression is a mature and voluntary defense occurring when unwanted feelings are consciously put aside and out of mind.

E. Projection, a less mature defense, involves unacceptable impulses being attributed to external sources.

3. B The cofactor that this patient is deficient in is vitamin B1 (thiamine). Given the patient's history, physical exam, and laboratory findings, he is probably suffering from alcohol withdrawal. It is known that alcoholics are at high risk for thiamine deficiency, given that they are often malnourished and that alcohol itself inhibits the absorption of thiamine. Some of the signs of thiamine deficiency include ataxia, nystagmus, and ophthalmoplegia (evidence of Wernicke's encephalopathy); confabulation and psychosis (indicating Korsakoff's psychosis); high-output cardiac failure (indicating wet beriberi); and peripheral neuropathy (indicating dry beriberi). The patient described has bilateral crackles in both lung fields, pitting edema of the extremities, and an enlarged heart on x-ray, all of which indicate heart failure. This patient also has evidence of Wernicke's encephalopathy (nystagmus and ophthalmoplegia) and peripheral neuropathy (wrist drop). Thiamine is used as a cofactor by three major enzymes: pyruvate dehydrogenase (PDH), alpha-ketoglutarate dehydrogenase (found in the TCA cycle), and transketolase. Transketolase is found in the hexose monophosphate shunt being involved in reactions which convert certain glycolytic intermediates (fructose 6-P and glyceraldehyde 3-P) into ribose 5-P, which is used in the synthesis of nucleotides.

A. Glycolysis does not contain the PDH enzyme.

C. The malate shuttle is involved in the aerobic conversion of cytoplasmic NADH (formed during glycolysis) into ATP. Of course, thiamine is not involved in any of these reactions.

D. Gluconeogenesis involves the conversion of certain amino acids, lactate, glycerol 3-phosphate, and fructose and galactose into glucose. Acetyl CoA cannot be used as a substrate and as such PDH is not used in gluconeogenesis, and again none of the enzymes involved in these pathways requires thiamine.

E. Fatty acid oxidation occurs in liver, muscle, and adipose tissue. None of the enzymes required in this process, from those needed to get fatty acids across the two membranes of the mitochondria to those within the mitochondrial matrix itself, requires thiamine as a cofactor.

4. B *Bordetella pertussis* is the causative agent of whooping cough. It is a gram negative coccobacillus that sensitizes the lungs to histamine leading to an explosive cough and also causes lymphocytosis. The DPT vaccine is effective in preventing whooping cough.

A. Respiratory syncytial virus is a major problem in the first year of life. It causes bronchiolitis and pneumonia but does not cause the characteristic cough.

C. *Haemophilus influenzae* causes meningitis, epiglottitis, bronchitis, pneumonia, and otitis media. It does not cause the histamine sensitization that leads to the characteristic cough in whooping cough disease.

D. *Streptococcus pneumoniae* is the commonest cause of bacterial lobar pneumonia.

E. *Legionella pneumophila* causes an atypical pneumonia or "walking" pneumonia. This is usually a progressive disease that is much more common in adults than children.

5. A The triad of arthritis, uveitis, and urethritis defines Reiter's syndrome. It is frequently associated with chlamydia infections (significance of sexual history) and HLA-B27 positive patients (significance of psoriasis and brother with AS). It is usually seen in young adult males.

B. Urethritis is not seen in psoriatic arthropathy.

C. Although the symptoms are similar, reactive arthritis is usually seen following GI infections (*Shigella, Salmonella, Helicobacter, Campylobacter, Yersinia*)

D. The arthritis in RA is chronic, not acute.

E. Urethritis is not seen in ankylosing spondylitis (AS) and the absence of sacroiliac joint inflammation precludes AS being the diagnosis.

6. B Rheumatoid arthritis is a chronic systemic disease that typically symmetrically affects joints. About 70% of patients will have a positive rheumatoid factor (antiglobulin antibodies) in blood. In this case, the patient has both rheumatoid arthritis and some type of renal disease that is causing her increased blood levels of creatinine and BUN. Methotrexate is an excellent choice for controlling the rheumatoid arthritis because it is not toxic to the kidneys.

A. Celecoxib is a cox-2 inhibitor. A cox-2 inhibitor will cause a decrease in prostaglandin production and a reduction in kidney perfusion that can lead to further kidney deterioration.

C. Indomethacin is not an ideal choice as it is a cox-1 inhibitor and will lead to further reduction in kidney perfusion.

D. Acetaminophen is a central cox inhibitor and will not reduce the inflammation in the periphery, although it will help with the pain.

E. Cyclosporine is an immunosuppressive drug and will probably do more harm than good. It could reduce the immune response enough to increase the chance of infections. Moreover, one of its major side effects is renal toxicity.

7. A Portal hypertension is most likely caused by cirrhosis of the liver in this man with a history of alcoholism. The clinical manifestations of portal hypertension include bleeding from gastroesophageal varices, splenomegaly, and dilation of periumbilical collateral vessels.

B. Increased central arterial pressure leads to increased risk for myocardial infarction or stroke, but not the findings in this patient.

C. Increased central venous pressure is usually a result of congestive heart failure and may present with shortness of breath and lower extremity edema.

D. This patient does not have signs or symptoms of increased pulmonary arterial pressure. Increased pulmonary arterial pressure occurs most often in response to increased pulmonary vascular resistance secondary to alveolar hypoxia.

8. D The most likely diagnosis is temporal arteritis. The vasculitis of temporal arteritis is usually granulomatous. The inner portion of the tunica media is affected, leading to granulomatous inflammation of the artery.

A. Vision is affected in approximately one-half of patients, with symptoms ranging from transient diplopia to blindness.

B. The pulmonary and cardiac vasculature is rarely affected in temporal arteritis.

C. The most commonly affected arteries are the temporal and ophthalmic.

E. Most patients with TA are females older than 50.

9. C *Helicobacter pylori* is an urease-positive curved bacteria. This is the causative agent responsible for most of the ulcers in the stomach and duodenum. The drug regimen given is used to eradicate *H. pylori*. An alternate regimen would be amoxicillin, clarithromycin, and omeprazole.

A. *Entamoeba histolytica* is a protozoan parasite that causes flasklike lesions in the colon and leads to dysentery.

B. The two most important *E. coli* are enterotoxigenic and enterohemorrhagic. The enterotoxigenic causes watery diarrhea and the enterohemorrhagic leads to dysentery.

D. *Salmonella typhi* causes ulcers in the terminal ileum and septicemia.

E. *Campylobacter jejuni* will cause partial mucosal invasion and is also a major cause of diarrhea.

10. D In this patient with renal hypoperfusion due to renal artery stenosis, the preservation of glomerular filtration is likely to be highly dependent on the actions of angiotensin II (which causes constriction of the efferent arteriole) and prostaglandins (which cause dilation of the afferent arteriole). ACE inhibitors, which interfere in the formation of angiotensin II, and cyclooxygenase inhibitors are thus contraindicated in patients with suspected renal hypoperfusion, as they may precipitate acute renal failure.

A. Hydralazine acts mainly to dilate arteries.

B. Metoprolol is a cardioselective beta-blocker.

C. Amlodipine is a dihydropyrimidine calcium channel blocker.

11. A The axillary nerve and the circumflex humeral artery are located at the surgical neck of the humerus. The axillary nerve (C5 and C6) innervates the deltoid muscle, and its interruption causes symptoms in this patient. The deltoid abducts, adducts, flexes, extends, and rotates arm medially. As the deltoid atrophies, the rounded contour of the shoulder would disappear. The circumflex humeral artery consists of an anterior and a posterior part, and they encircle the surgical neck of the humerus.

B. The subscapular artery is the largest branch of the axillary artery, and it divides into the thoracodorsal and circumflex scapular arteries.

C. The thoracoacromial artery is a short trunk of the axillary artery and has pectoral, clavicular, acromial, and deltoid branches.

D. The axillary artery becomes the brachial artery at the inferior border of the teres major muscle.

E. The subclavian artery becomes the axillary artery at the lateral border of the first rib.

12. C The patient has galactosemia, which is most often due to an inherited, autosomal recessive defect in galactose 1-phosphate uridyl transferase, which converts galactose-1-phosphate into UDP-galactose, which can then be used as a carbon source for glycolysis or gluconeogenesis. This defect results in toxic accumulation of substances such as galactitol, because galactose cannot be properly metabolized. Cataracts, hepatomegaly, and mental retardation are common symptoms. (A smaller percentage of cases have been reported with inherited mutations in galactokinase.)

A. Aldolase B defects result in severe hypoglycemia secondary to fructose-1-phosphate accumulation.

B. While lactase deficiency can produce diarrhea after milk consumption, toxicity is not a common manifestation.

D. Fructokinase deficiency is benign and asymptomatic, with fructosuria an incidental finding.

E. Glucose-6-phosphate dehydrogenase deficiency leads to hemolytic anemia when patients undergo stressors (infections or particular medications such as anti-malarial compounds).

13. A Anticonvulsant phenytoin, Dilantin, decreases seizure activity by stabilizing neuronal membranes via decreasing influx/increasing efflux of sodium ions in the motor cortex during nerve impulse generation.

B. Phenytoin is clinically used for grand mal seizures, status epilepticus, and complex partial seizures. It may actually increase the frequency of petit mal, or absence, seizures.

C. Phenytoin is an *inducer* of CYP1a2, 3A3/4, and 3A5-7.

D. The classic sign is gingival hyperplasia.

E. This drug is categorized as Category D, considered unsafe. Common teratogenic effects are cardiac abnormalities.

14. B REM sleep is termed "paradoxical sleep" because it has the same EEG waveform pattern as the awake, alert, and actively concentrating state (beta). Beta waves are characterized by high frequency and low amplitude.

A. Roughly 25% of sleep is spent in REM sleep. The length of REM sleep decreases with age.

C. Serotonin is the neurotransmitter important for sleep initiation. Acetylcholine is the primary neurotransmitter involved in REM sleep.

D. Dreaming occurs in REM sleep.

E. Imipramine, a tricyclic antidepressant, decreases stage 4 sleep and is helpful in treating enuresis (bed-wetting) for this reason.

15. C Patients with severe chronic bronchitis, which can be exacerbated by common infections, are often-times called "blue bloaters" due to their cyanotic and edematous appearance. Chronic bronchitis patients have a low partial oxygen pressure (PaO_2) due to ventilation/perfusion mismatch and hypoventilation. This hypoventilation leads to chronic hypercapnia, hypoxemia, and respiratory acidosis. This retention of CO_2 and subsequent acidosis leads to a right shift of the oxygen-hemoglobin dissociation curve. A normal PaO_2 ranges from 80 to 100 mm Hg with normal saturation from 90% to 100%. You should be familiar with a few of the normal standard values on this curve. When PaO_2 is 95 mm Hg, O_2 saturation is approximately 97%. When PaO_2 is 60 mm Hg, O_2 saturation is approximately 90%. When PaO_2 is 40 mm Hg, O_2 saturation is approximately 75%. When PaO_2 is 25 mm Hg, O_2 saturation is approximately 50%. In a normal oxygen-hemoglobin dissociation curve the steep slope of the curve begins around a PaO_2 of 60 mm Hg. This is when the percent saturation begins to rapidly fall with small decreases in PaO_2. PaO_2 of 90, 80, 60, and 50 all have percent saturations that would be expected and reflect only minor changes. The only answer that represents a right shift in the curve and shows a dramatic decrease in percent saturation is a PaO_2 of 70 with a percent saturation of hemoglobin of 60. Since we know that a PaO_2 of 60 mm Hg should have an approximate percent saturation of 90, we can immediately be alerted to the answer's values as being abnormal.

A, B, D, E. All represent a normal oxygen-hemoglobin dissociation curve without shift.

16. B Schiller-Duval bodies are the characteristic cell of a endodermal sinus (yolk sac) tumor. These tumors secrete alpha-fetoprotein, which can also be stained for histologically by immunoperoxidase techniques.

A. Beta-HCG is secreted by choriocarcinomas.

C. Estrogen is secreted by granulosa cell tumors.

D. Androgens are secreted by Sertoli-Leydig cell tumors.

E. Thyroid hormone is secreted by struma ovarii tumors, a subtype of a specialized, monodermal mature teratoma.

17. E Cromolyn sodium is used to stabilize the cell membranes of mast cells to prevent the release of histamine. It is only indicated in chronic use as a preventive medicine. It has no indication for use in acute attacks of asthma.

A. Ipratropium is an anti-cholinergic agent used to prevent bronchoconstriction by the parasympathetic system.

B. Albuterol is used to dilate the bronchioles.

C. Magnesium is used to relax the smooth muscles of the bronchioles.

D. Prednisone, although not fast acting, is indicated in a severe acute attack of asthma to reduce inflammation and reduce the chance of subsequent attacks in the acute phase. It is given as a high-dose burst for four or five days and stopped without tapering. The onset of relief from prednisone is approximately 12 hours after the first dose.

18. C This child likely has kwashiorkor, a disease of selective protein malnutrition found in regions of famine and recurrent diarrheal illness. It is characterized by lethargy, fatty liver, and edema.

A. Inadequate vitamin C consumption leads to scurvy, a disorder of collagen synthesis characterized by bleeding gums and easy bruising.

B. Inadequate vitamin D consumption leads to rickets, characterized by bowing of long bones due to inadequate bone mineralization.

D. Decreased fat consumption will not lead to the symptoms described.

19. D Extension of the forearm at the elbow occurs via the radial nerve and triceps muscle, a lower trunk derivation. All other actions and sensation travel through the upper trunk.

A, B, C, E. These actions occur via the upper trunk.

20. C Psychological testing can be broadly divided into two categories—objective and projective tests. Objective tests typically provide numerical scores and patterns that can be statistically analyzed; they are generally pencil and paper tests. Projective tests are less black and white, as they purposefully introduce ambiguity, which requires individuals to use more interpretation and is more dependent on emotional and psychological factors than objective testing. The MMPI (now in its updated version MMPI-2) is a self-report inventory that is the most researched and used personality assessment tool.

A, B, D, E. The TAT is a projective test.

21. B *Staph saprophyticus* is a gram positive coccus that is catalase positive, but coagulase negative. It is the second most common causative agent of urinary tract infections in young sexually active women.

A. *Staph aureus* is rarely a cause of UTIs and is coagulase positive.
C. *Strep faecalis* is catalase negative.
D. *E. coli*, although the most common cause of UTIs in women, is gram negative.
E. *Neisseria gonorrhoeae* is gram negative. It is not a common cause of UTIs in women.

22. C This patient is suffering from Parkinson's disease. Chlorpromazine (Thorazine) is a dopamine antagonist and will worsen the symptoms of Parkinson's disease.

A. Amantadine is an antiviral agent used to treat influenza infection that also has shown efficacy in the treatment of Parkinson's disease.
B. Bromocriptine is a dopamine agonist that is used in the treatment of Parkinson's disease.
D. Levodopa/carbidopa is used in the treatment of Parkinson's disease. Levodopa is a dopamine precursor that crosses the blood-brain barrier and increases levels of dopamine in the substantia nigra. It is compounded with carbidopa to limit the amount of peripheral conversion to dopamine, which lessens the necessary dose as well as diminishing side effects.

E. Pergolide is a dopamine agonist that is used in the treatment of Parkinson's disease.
F. Selegiline is a MAO-B inhibitor that slows the degradation of dopamine and is used in the treatment of Parkinson's disease.
G. Tolcapone is a member of a new class of drugs (the COMT inhibitors) used in the treatment of Parkinson's disease. They act by inhibiting the degradation of both dopamine and levodopa.
H. Trihexyphenidyl is an anticholinergic used as adjunctive treatment of Parkinson's disease, mainly for tremor. This class of drugs acts by decreasing the increased CNS cholinergic tone that results from the depletion of striatal dopamine.

23. B Medications that irreversibly inhibit the parietal cell H^+, K^+-ATPase, often called proton pump inhibitors, potently inhibit all phases of gastric acid secretion. Since they act at the final common pathway of all stimuli to acid secretion, these are by far the most effective antisecretory drugs.

A. Although H_2 blockers are effective in reducing gastric acid secretion, they only inhibit one of several stimuli to acid secretion.
C. Acetylcholine is only one of several stimuli to gastric acid secretion; no medications that act at the acetylcholine receptors are used because of side effects.
D. Gastrin receptors are only one of several stimuli for gastric acid secretion; currently no drugs exist that act at the gastrin receptor.

24. C Major depressive disorder, which has a lifetime prevalence of between 8 and 12%, is approximately twice as common in women as compared to men.

A. Bipolar disorder is thought to be equally prevalent in males and females. There is no history of manic episodes.
B. Autistic disorder is more common in boys and results in inability to function in society.
D. Schizophrenia is thought to be equally prevalent in males and females. There is no evidence of thought disorder in this woman.
E. Attention deficit disorder (ADD) is thought to be more common in boys and does not present in this way. There is usually a lifelong history of inability to concentrate, usually with some degree of hyperactivity.

25. D The patient has iatrogenic Cushing's syndrome from high-dose corticosteroid treatment for systemic lupus erythematosus. Cushing's syndrome is associated with obesity, which tends to be centrally located and can also be redistributed to the face. Hypertension, especially with diastolic hypertension, proximal muscle weakness, and elevated fasting blood glucose levels from insulin resistance are all findings associated with Cushing's syndrome. However, the most common cause of hypercortisolism is iatrogenic, particularly when using corticosteroids to treat autoimmune diseases. High-dose corticosteroid therapy may be required in any number of inflammatory conditions such as SLE and it is the standard of care practice to gradually reduce the patient's dose to the minimum required to control the symptoms and signs of the disease, as well as reduce the side effects of therapy.

A. Although an appropriate test to help distinguish between Cushing's disease, Cushing's syndrome, and ectopic ACTH-secreting tumor, it is not the best choice since the patient has SLE and is being treated with steroids.
B. The patient is not a diabetic and has no history of diabetes. Iatrogenically induced Cushing's syndrome may cause insulin resistance.
C. Another appropriate test that is used in conjunction with a dexamethasone suppression test for evaluating endogenous Cushing's syndrome, but not the most appropriate answer.
E. Although not very specific, it may be ordered to evaluate for pituitary adenoma in Cushing's disease. It is not the correct answer in this scenario.

26. C Small cell carcinoma of the lung is not amenable to surgical resection but is sensitive to radiation and chemotherapy, with cure rates of 15 to 25%.

A. Surgery is the treatment of choice for non-small cell cancers of respectable dimensions.
B. Surgery is appropriate unless there are extra thoracic metastases, phrenic or laryngeal nerve palsy, or involvement of the esophagus or pericardium.
D. Surgery is appropriate when possible.
E. A hamartoma is a benign mass of disorganized, but mature, tissue that can be easily resected.

27. C Hepatitis C is commonly transmitted by needle sticks. There is no vaccine available for prevention. Patients with hepatitis C often progress to liver failure.

A. The transmission of hepatitis A is oral-fecal, not needle sticks. There is a separate vaccine available for hepatitis A.
B. The presence of anti-HBs antibodies indicates immunity to this hepatitis. There is a vaccine for this virus.
D. Hepatitis D requires the presence of hepatitis B virus to enter the cells. This student's immunity to hepatitis B also protects him from this virus. There is no vaccine for this virus.
E. Transmission of this virus is generally oral-fecal. There is no vaccine for this virus.

28. C This patient had been well controlled with a beta-agonist (albuterol) for several years. Now she is having exacerbations and the beta-agonist is no longer enough. The standard protocol for an asthmatic who is not well controlled on beta-agonists is to add an inhaled steroid such as fluticasone that is taken regularly. The beta-agonist should continue to be used for acute attacks.

A. This is no longer sufficient. The patient needs an additional agent to control her asthma.
B. While it is necessary to add fluticasone, the albuterol cannot be discontinued. It is necessary to overcome bronchospasm during acute attacks.
D. Ipratropium is a vagal inhibitor that results in bronchodilation, resulting in a similar affect as the beta-agonists. However, it has a slower onset and lower effect in most asthmatics, so it is not one of the first-line agents for asthma. It is used commonly in COPD patients.
E. Leukotriene inhibitors are newer agents, sometimes used to treat asthma. However, these would only be used if inhaled steroids were insufficient or not tolerated. They are also used in aspirin-sensitive asthmatics.

29. C In an anterior myocardial infarction, the main artery supplying the myocardium is the left anterior descending artery. For an anterior myocardial infarction, the diagnostic leads are the anterior chest leads V1-V6.

A. The RCA and its early branches supply the majority of the blood to the right atrium and right ventricle. In a myocardial infarction of the RCA, the diagnostic leads are II, III, and aVF and it may also involve the PDA.

B. The LAD supplies blood to the left atria and the posterior aspect of the left ventricle. In a myocardial infarction of the LAD, the diagnostic leads are either the anterolateral leads I, aVL, V5, and V6 or the lateral leads I, aVL, and V1-V6.

D. The PDA is the largest branch off the right main coronary artery. The PDA typically supplies part of the interventricular septum.

E. The thoracoacromial artery is not part of coronary circulation. The axillary artery gives off the thoracoacromial artery, which branches and supplies portions of the shoulder girdle including the pectoral and deltoid regions.

30. D The binding of oxygen at any given heme group produces so-called cooperative, or increased, binding of oxygen at the rest of the heme groups of the molecule, thus allowing hemoglobin to deliver more oxygen to the tissues even when the changes in partial oxygen pressure are minimal.

A. Carbon dioxide binding to amino groups of hemoglobin stabilize the T deoxy form and decrease the affinity for oxygen.

B. Fetal hemoglobin (HbF) has significantly greater affinity for oxygen than HbA. This is due to HbF's weak binding to 2,3 BPG.

C. Hemoglobin is a tetramer that binds one molecule of 2,3 BPG.

E. Bohr's effect, since carbon dioxide binding to hemoglobin decreases pH, thus decreasing the affinity of hemoglobin for oxygen.

31. D The patient shows signs of hyperthyroidism, and the most common cause of hyperthyroidism is Graves' disease, which is far more common in females. Other signs include Graves' ophthalmopathy, dermopathy, nervousness, increased appetite, tremor, warm and moist skin, and emotional lability. Due to unknown mechanisms, T lymphocytes become sensitized to thyroid antigens and stimulate B cells to produce antibodies. The thyroid stimulating immunoglobulin of the IgG class bind to the thyrotropin receptors on the thyroid glands and stimulate the production of T3 and T4.

A. T3 and T4 are made from iodine. Thyroid follicles trap inorganic iodide and transport it against a concentration gradient by a Na/I symporter. Iodine is then oxidized by peroxidase.

B. Thyroid deiodinase releases free iodine from T3/T4 in peripheral tissues. Since the kidney can excrete the free iodine, both the kidney and the thyroid compete for iodine in the circulation.

C. Thyroglobulin is a glycoprotein backbone to which T3 and T4 are attached during thyroid hormone synthesis.

E is incorrect.

32. C His total cholesterol is mildly elevated above the desired level of 200. His HDL is only mildly below the desired level of 35, but his triglycerides are substantially elevated. Gemfibrozil is effective at reducing triglycerides and mildly increasing HDL. This would create the appropriate effect in this patient whose main problem is high triglycerides.

A. Simvastatin is a HMG-CoA reductase inhibitor and is most effective at lowering LDL. This patient's LDL is well within the normal and desired range, and simvastatin is not needed.

B. Niacin is primarily used to raise HDL, although it also reduces LDL. Although this patient has mildly decreased HDL, niacin would not address the high triglycerides as well as gemfibrozil. It also has unpleasant side effects, such as flushing.

D. Cholestyramine is a bile-acid resin that binds bile acids in the intestine and prevents reabsorption. This forces the liver to use more cholesterol. It reduces LDL; however, it is known to increase triglycerides, so it is inappropriate in this case.

E is incorrect.

33. E
A The polypeptide capsule of *B. anthracis* provides antiphagocytic properties to the organism, and antibodies directed against the capsule do not provide protection.

B. Edema factor is a component of anthrax toxin. When combined with the protective antigen component of anthrax toxin, it is observed to cause edema in laboratory animals.

C. Shiga-like toxin is not produced by *B. anthracis*. Shiga-like toxin is produced via a plasmid carried by the *Shigella* species and by *E. coli*. It inhibits protein synthesis and causes cell death within the gastrointestinal tract and can cause a severe, although self-limited, diarrhea.

D. Lethal factor is the third component of anthrax toxin. The combination of lethal factor with the protective antigen component of anthrax toxin causes death.

34. E This patient best characterizes histrionic personality disorder, a Cluster B personality disorder (the "dramatic" cluster) that is derived from the older diagnosis, hysteria. There are several diagnostic criteria for this disorder, but key points are a need to be the center of attention, rapidly shifting and shallow emotions, and excessive concern over appearance.

A. Borderline personality is also a Cluster B disorder, although it is more characterized by unstable interpersonal relationships, poor anger control, and frequent thoughts of suicide or self-harm behaviors (cutting themselves).

B. Narcissistic personality is a Cluster C disorder (the "anxious" cluster) characterized by grandiosity (extreme arrogance and self-importance), a need for excessive admiration, and a lack of empathy for others.

C. Dependent personality is a Cluster C disorder diagnosed when individuals exhibit a pattern of excessive need to be taken care of, for others to make decisions for them, and for much reassurance from others to make decisions for their own life.

D. Paranoid personality is a Cluster A disorder (the "odd cluster") characterized by excessive distrust and suspiciousness of others, difficulty confiding in others, and tendency to hold grudges.

35. D Rheumatic fever is a common cause of AV valve insufficiency due to complications of group A *Streptococcus pyogenes* pharyngitis. The presentation of rheumatic fever includes a history of a self-limiting sore throat, but the immunologic reaction of the bacterial infection causes late onset of symptoms. The diagnosis of rheumatic fever includes the presence of two major Jones criteria (carditis, polyarthritis, Sydenham chorea, erythema marginatum, subcutaneous nodules) or one major and two minor criteria (fever, polyarthralgias, previous acute rheumatic fever, elevated ESR or C-reactive protein or leukocytosis, prolonged PR interval) in conjunction with evidence of a preceding *Streptococcal* infection.

A. The AV valve in the right ventricle is called the tricuspid valve. The AV valve in the left ventricle is called the bicuspid or mitral valve. It is commonly damaged in rheumatic heart disease.

B. Infection of *Staphylococcus aureus* is mostly seen with tricuspid valve damage. Because of venous return to the right ventricles, tricuspid valve damage commonly occurs in IV drug users.

C & E are incorrect. See above.

36. E Whipple disease is a rare, systemic condition principally affecting the intestine, central nervous system, and joints. Skin hyperpigmentation is a "red flag" for this disease. Whipple occurs more commonly in white males in their 30s to 40s. The diagnosis rests on light microscopic changes of PAS-positive macrophages, which contain rod-shaped bacilli *Tropheryma whippelii* by electron microscopy. Inflammation, however, is absent at affected sites.

A. The pathology describes a destructive process commonly seen in pseudomembranous colitis caused by *Clostridium difficile*.

B. The pathology describes inflammation commonly seen in celiac sprue due to gluten sensitivity.

C. The pathology describes inflammation and destruction commonly seen in patients with Crohn's disease and ulcerative colitis.

D. The pathology describes mucosa destruction commonly seen in patients with ulcerative colitis.

37. D Captopril, an ACE inhibitor, has cough as one of its side effects. Other side effects are rash, neutropenia, angioedema, and hyperkalemia.

A. Increased energy is almost never a "side effect."

B. Psychogenic medications such as some SSRIs may decrease sex drive.

C. Diuretics cause increased volume and frequency of urination.

E. On the exam, trust yourself. If you don't recall the option at all from one of your classes, it is probably the wrong answer, as is the case here.

38. E

A. Since they lack the ability to replicate independent of a host, viruses must be infectious in order to survive in nature.

B. Viruses are not living organisms.

C. A viral genome may be RNA or DNA, but not both.

D. Some viruses are surrounded by a membrane composed of glycoproteins, proteins, and lipids. This membrane is called an envelope.

39. C SSRI antidepressants have the lowest side effect profile of all of the antidepressants and so they are the first line in treating depression in the elderly.

A. Amitriptyline is a tricyclic antidepressant. TCAs are especially problematic in the elderly due to their anticholinergic and antiadrenergic side effects (urinary retention and orthostatic hypotension respectively are the most worrisome in the geriatric population).

B. Olanzapine is an atypical antipsychotic. This patient has no psychotic symptoms.

D. Tranylcypromine is a MAOI. While they do not have the anticholinergic side effect profile of the TCAs, they are not first-line agents due to their drug-drug and food interactions.

E. While ECT is used for depression, it is reserved for intractable cases, psychotic depression, or the severely incapacitated patient.

40. A The question is really asking you about p450 enzymes and which drugs interact with them. Cimetidine is known to cause gynecomastia in some males. It inhibits the p450 enzymes of the liver, thus estrogen hormones remain active longer and cause gynecomastia.

B. Phenytoin induces p450 enzymes.

C. Carbamazepine also induces p450 enzymes.

D. Calcium channel blockers neither induce nor inhibit p450 enzymes.

E. Quinidine is metabolized by p450 enzymes, it does not inhibit or induce it.

41. E This patient is suffering from hyperthyroidism, also called Graves' disease. In hyperthyroidism, the TSH (thyroid stimulating hormone) is low due to the negative feedback loop of thyroid hormone. Treatment is medical or radio ablation. After radiotherapy, many patients become hypothyroid and must take daily supplemental thyroid hormone.

A. TSH is elevated in hypothyroidism, not hyperthyroidism.

B. Thyroid carcinoma usually presents with an enlarged thyroid gland or as a thyroid nodule. There are not usually signs of hyperthyroidism. The incidence of thyroid cancers is very low, accounting for less than 1% of all malignancies.

C. Although thyroid adenomas are more prevalent than thyroid carcinoma, they are still rare and do not usually result in hyperthyroid symptoms.

D. Hashimoto's thyroiditis is associated with hypothyroidism.

42. D This is a classic presentation for meningococcal meningitis. The headache, photophobia, and meningismus make meningitis the most likely diagnosis, and the LP finding of PMN predominance, low glucose, and high protein make it likely to be a bacterial meningitis. The rash on the legs of this patient is the classic sign of a meningococcal infection, and this type of meningitis is also found in crowded areas such as college dorms.

A. Pneumococcal meningitis presents similarly, but there is no rash.

B. *Staphylococcus aureus* meningitis usually occurs in the hospital due to neurosurgery or because of trauma that directly introduces the bacteria to the site.

C. *Listeria* meningitis occurs in immunocompromised patients such as neonates, elderly, or AIDS patients.

E. *Streptococcus agalactiae* is a bacteria that is transferred to neonates from their mothers in the birth canal and, thus, causes meningitis in infants.

43. D For the diagnosis of anorexia nervosa, a person's body weight must fall below 85% of the ideal body weight for that person. This patient's current weight does not meet the criteria, because 85% of her ideal body weight is 102 pounds.

A. Up to 50% of patients with anorexia nervosa binge and purge.

B. Amenorrhea in postmenarchal females is part of the diagnostic criteria for the diagnosis of anorexia nervosa.

C. Anorexia nervosa is more common in higher socioeconomic classes.

E. More than 90% of patients diagnosed with anorexia nervosa are female.

44. B Efficacy is the ability of two or more drugs to produce the same, specific result regardless of differences in amounts of drug prescribed. A good example is opioids—regardless of different dosages required they all produce the same effect.

A. Potency is related to the amount of drug necessary to reach an effect. In the example above, drug B has more potency than drug A, because it takes half as much to reach the same effect.

C. Effective dose is the amount of drug necessary to reach the desired effect.

D. LD_{50} is the amount of drug necessary to be lethal in 50% of subjects.

45. C These are the two most common causes of cervicitis and are both treated simultaneously. *N. gonorrhoea* is a gram negative nonencapsulated, oxidase-positive diplococci that does not ferment maltose. Chlamydia is determined by fluorescent antibody stain, looking for any cytoplasmic inclusions.

A. There is no mention of any painful genital ulcers. You would use the Tzanck smear to confirm diagnosis since this is a virus and a gram stain would not show anything.
B. Usually the patient has a scant vaginal discharge that looks like cottage cheese. Since this is a yeast, KOH preparation would be used to arrive at this diagnosis.
D. A protozoan that you need to diagnosis on wet mount.
E. Patient does not mention any foul "fishy" malodorous odor that is intensified when KOH is added to discharge.

46. C The loss of two of the α-globin genes results in a mild microcytic anemia without hemolysis and no dependence on transfusion. The loss of the two alleles can come from either losing one gene on each chromosome or both from the same chromosome. The phenotypes will remain indistinguishable.

A. The α-globin gene is normal.
B. The loss of only one gene makes the person a carrier of the trait with no symptoms.
D. The loss of all but one α-globin gene is hemoglobin H, which is manifested by hemolysis and anemia.
E. The loss of all of the α-globin genes causes hydrops fetalis and results in severe anemia and death in utero.

47. A Colchicine is one of the medications used to treat gout, a disease caused by high levels of uric acid in the blood. Colchicine decreases the movement of granulocytes to the affected area by causing the depolymerization of tubulin. It also inhibits the synthesis and release of leukotrienes.

B. This is the mechanism of action of allopurinol, also used in the treatment of gout.
C. This is the mechanism of action of uricosuric agents such as Probenecid and sulfinpyrazone used in the treatment of gout.
D. This is the mechanism of aspirin, not used in the treatment of gout.
E. This would be the mechanism of an antibiotic, used in the treatment of cellulitis, not gout.

48. E Cystic fibrosis is an autosomal recessive disease caused by a mutation in the CFTR (cystic fibrosis transmembrane conductance regulator) gene. CF is the most common genetic disorder in white Americans, occurring in about 1 per 3400 births. Newborns often show the signs of CF by having meconium ileus, volvulus, or other gastrointestinal problems. Then, patients experience chronic cough and recurrent respiratory tract infections. As respiratory function continues to decline, pulmonary function tests reveal hypoxemia and decreases in forced vital capacity (FVC) and forced expiratory volume in one second (FEV1). As a result of the pulmonary manifestations, the chest x-ray often shows hyperinflation with bronchial changes secondary to chronic inflammation. The sweat test reveals an increase in the amount of chloride in sweat in CF patients.

A, B, C, D. See **E** above.

49. B Prevalence ratio is defined as the total number of individuals in the population who have a disease divided by the total population. The total number of individuals with the disease in 2001 is 150 and the total population is 3000.

A. 50/1600 is the number of individuals newly diagnosed with the disease divided by the total number of men in this population.
C. 50/3000 is the incident rate of the disease. Incident rate is defined as the number of new individuals who develop a disease divided by the total number of individuals at risk for the disease during a given time period.
D. 150/1400 is the total number of individuals who have the disease divided by the total number of women in this population.
E. 50/1400 is the number of individuals newly diagnosed with the disease divided by the total number of women in this population.

50. E Due to blood loss and subsequent transfusion with PRBC only, the patient is extremely low on clotting factors. Fresh frozen plasma (FFP) has clotting factors to replace the ones lost.

A. RBCs alone with no FFP will further dilute the remaining clotting factors.
B. Anaphylaxis to transfusions occurs immediately, not hours after start of transfusion.
C. There is no indication to use heparin on this patient who is low on clotting factors.
D. Vitamin K would have no immediate effect.

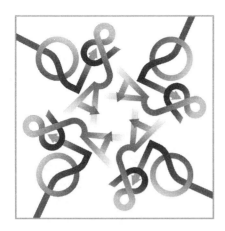

QUESTIONS BLOCK 2

51. A 25-year-old male is involved in a motor vehicle accident and presents with severe abdominal and chest pain, shortness of breath, and dyspnea. Chest x-rays reveal large intestine in the left thorax consistent with rupture of the left hemidiaphragm. Which of the following statements is true regarding the diaphragm?

A. Ruptures of the diaphragm are equally likely to occur on the right and left sides.

B. The celiac artery branches from the aorta before the aorta passes through the diaphragm.

C. Neither the right nor left phrenic nerves actually pass through the diaphragm.

D. The motor supply of the diaphragm arises from the ventral roots of C2-C4.

E. The main arteries that supply the diaphragm are the phrenic arteries and two branches of the internal thoracic artery.

52. A 55-year-old married male CEO has been with the same company for 15 years. He feels that there is nothing to be accomplished at his current company and is bored with what he is doing. His wife of 30 years is engaged in social activities and clubs. Their children are no longer living at home. He has been paying attention to his 35-year-old secretary, a former model. He is most likely experiencing changes associated with which of Erikson's stages?

A. Industry vs. inferiority

B. Ego integrity vs. despair

C. Initiative vs. guilt

D. Generativity vs. self-absorption

E. Autonomy vs. shame and doubt

53. A patient comes to your office stating that he wishes to fast for one week for religious purposes. He is allowing himself to drink water, but will not be eating any food during this time period. He also tells you that he has a known deficiency in hepatic glucose 6-phosphatase (von Gierke's disease). Based upon this information, from which of the following metabolic processes would his brain derive most of its energy after the first 24 hours of fasting?

A. Protein catabolism

B. Gluconeogenesis

C. Glycogenolysis

D. Ketogenesis

E. The brain would have no source of energy available

54. A 40-year old-female immigrant from Mexico comes to your office for a physical for her work. She states that she is PPD positive but does not have an active infection. Which of the following statements is true concerning *Mycobacterium tuberculosis*?

A. The BCG vaccine is widely used in the United States to prevent *M. tuberculosis* infection.

B. PPD test indicates an active ongoing infection.

C. TB is most commonly transmitted by the exchange of fluids.

D. The initial infection of *M. tuberculosis* is in the apical part of the lungs.

E. *M. tuberculosis* is best grown on Lowenstein-Jensen medium.

55. A 35-year-old white male presents with dyspepsia. A further evaluation reveals guaiac-positive stools and multiple ulcers in the fundic region of the stomach. What pharmacological approach would you use in treating this patient?

A. Sucralfate with an antacid

B. Metoclopramide

C. Fexofenadine

D. Diphenoxylate

E. Omeprazole

56. A 62-year-old male smoker and alcoholic presents to the ER complaining of four months of worsening dysphagia. Work-up reveals a mass that is found to be an esophageal adenocarcinoma. **See Figure 56.** Which of the following applies best?

A. Esophageal adenocarcinoma is usually preceded by a columnar to squamous metaplasia of the esophageal epithelium.

B. Smoking and alcohol have been shown not to increase the risk of any type of esophageal cancer.

C. Adenocarcinoma of the esophagus tends to metastasize early due to the lack of serosa in the esophagus.

D. Long-standing reflux does not predispose one to develop Barrett's esophagus.

E. Esophagitis, a risk factor from development of Barrett's esophagus, is not a potential consequence of a sliding esophageal hernia.

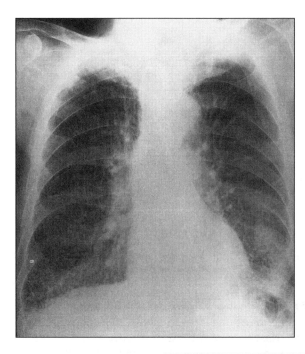

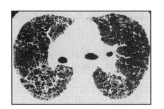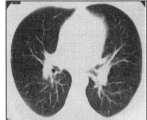

Figure 57 Reproduced with permission from Armstrong. Diagnostic Imaging, 4/e. Blackwell Science, Ltd., 1998.

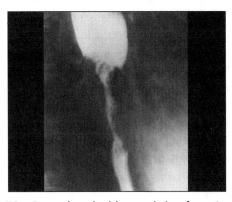

Figure 56 Reproduced with permission from Armstrong. Diagnostic Imaging, 4/e. Blackwell Science, Ltd., 1998.

57. A 68-year-old man with a 50-pack-per-year smoking history presents with increasing shortness of breath and a nonproductive cough. Physical examination is remarkable for diffuse inspiratory crackles and lack of lower extremity edema. A chest radiograph shows diffuse ground glass opacities. **(See Figure 57.)** Pulmonary function testing shows a markedly decreased total lung capacity (TLC) and an increased ratio of forced expiratory volume in one second to forced vital capacity (FEV_1/FVC). This man is most likely to have which of the following diseases?

A. Asthma

B. Emphysema

C. Idiopathic pulmonary fibrosis

D. Chronic bronchitis

58. On leaving your shift, one of your last duties to report to the oncoming physician is that your patient in room 12 is having some problems with his vision and a headache. The patient was admitted the previous night with the diagnosis of diabetic ketoacidosis. On coming to work the next day, you find the patient had emergency surgery for an infection which required a large debridement of his left frontal sinus. You also see that he is now receiving Amphotericin B. You recognize that your patient's headache and vision changes were most likely caused by:

A. *Staph aureus*

B. *Pseudomonas aeruginosa*

C. *Clostridium perfringens*

D. *Aspergillus*

E. Mucor

59. A known substance abuser comes to your substance abuse program. After taking a detailed history you are not concerned about this patient displaying tolerance or withdrawal to which of the following substances?

A. Nicotine

B. Alcohol

C. Caffeine

D. PCP

E. Benzodiazepines

60. A 19-year-old male, who lives in a dormitory at the local college, presents to your clinic complaining of a severe headache and mild fever associated with an intractable "hacking" cough. He describes chest soreness, which he believes to be due to his relentless coughing. He denies sputum production. Chest exam reveals symmetrical expansion with respirations, no wheezes, mild bilateral basilar crackles, and no changes in tactile fremitus. Dermatologic exam reveals multiple erythematous plaques with a "target" or "iris" morphology. Chest x-ray demonstrates reticulonodular morphology in both lower lobes of the lung, indicative of interstitial infiltration.

Which of the following is true concerning the organism responsible for this patient's symptoms?

A. It's cell wall lacks muramic acid, and thus the organism cannot be seen upon Gram's stain.

B. It is an obligate intracellular bacteria.

C. It is a gram-negative diplococcus, also known for causing otitis media in adults.

D. Air-conditioning water cooling tanks serve as one of its reservoirs.

E. It requires cholesterol for *in vitro* culture.

61. Which of the following best pairs a potential toxin and its appropriate treatment/antidote?

A. Lead/Penicillamine

B. Streptokinase/Dimercaprol

C. Opioids/Ethanol

D. Warfarin/Protamine

E. Benzodiazepines/Flumazenil

62. A 65-year-old woman presents to her gynecologist complaining of "something falling out of my vagina." Exam reveals severe uterine prolapse. The decision is made to perform a total abdominal hysterectomy. Which of the following statements is true regarding uterine and related anatomy?

A. The uterine arteries are direct branches of the aorta.

B. The main blood supply of the uterus travels in the round ligament.

C. The broad ligament functions primarily in support of the uterus.

D. The ovarian arteries are branches of the uterine artery.

E. During ligation of the uterine arteries the ureters are at a high risk of being damaged.

63. A 26-year-old male law student presents to his primary care physician's office with the complaint of having more than four bowel movements a day. They have been accompanied by severe cramping and mucus. His visit has been precipitated by the fact that yesterday he passed a gross amount of bright red blood per rectum. Over the past 18 months he has been increasingly fatigued and has lost about 10 pounds, things that he has attributed to stress as a law student. Barium enema shows loss of haustrations and colonoscopy shows hemorrhaging, mucosal erythema, and gross ulcerations which are continuous in nature. Based on this, the expected pathology report and surgical outcome would be:

A. Transmural inflammatory involvement of the bowel with noncaseating granulomas and fissures exhibiting skipping phenomena. Surgical prognosis poor.

B. Transmural inflammatory involvement of the bowel with noncaseating granulomas and fissures exhibiting skipping phenomena. Surgical prognosis good.

C. Diffuse superficial ulceration extending to the muscularis mucosa, no involvement of the serosa, marked polyp formation. Surgical prognosis good.

D. Neutrophilic infiltration of the muscularis only. Surgical prognosis good.

E. Small spherical outpouchings of atrophic mucosa with absent muscularis propria alongside the taenia coli. Surgical outcome poor.

64. Which of the following hemoglobin dissociation curves would be expected in someone who has been vigorously exercising for an hour? **See Figure 64.**

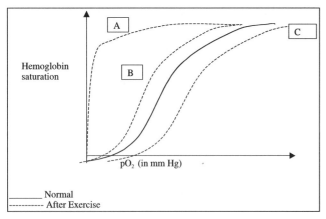

Figure 64

65. A 30-year-old female comes to the ER with a sudden onset of violent nausea and vomiting. She relates she had been out earlier in the evening and had three glasses of wine with dinner. She is currently on five different medications. Of the five medications, which one is the most likely cause of her vomiting:

A. Tetracycline for her acne

B. Propranolol for heart palpitations

C. Buspirone for anxiety

D. Diphenhydramine for allergic rhinitis

E. Metronidazole for a vaginal infection

66. You see an infant in the grocery store with her father. Having just studied developmental milestones and after having observed the child briefly, you estimate her age to be 8 months. Assuming normal development, this would most accurately be based on which observation:

A. You hear the infant "cooing"

B. She brings her hands to midline

C. Social smile

D. Ability to hold head up steadily

E. She cries and clings to father as strangers pass by

67. A 38-year-old male presents to your clinic complaining of chronic hematuria. He has recently immigrated to the United States from Egypt. He states that this has been an ongoing problem since childhood, and recalls comparing the color of his urinary stream with that of other boys (hematuria

being quite common). Your urological consultation reports that this patient has a bladder carcinoma, and suggests the following etiology:

A. Chronic *E. coli* urinary tract infection

B. Repeated untreated acute urinary tract infections with *E. coli*

C. Infection with adenovirus serotype 11

D. Chronic infection with *Schistosoma mansoni*

E. Chronic infection with *Schistosoma haematobium*

68. A 20-year-old previously healthy male house cleaner presented with new-onset fatigue, jaundice, and shortness of breath after spending a day cleaning the home of an eccentric owner who would put mothflakes under all her rugs. Work-up of the patient revealed a hemolytic anemia. An extensive family history was obtained by the attending physician after the patient's mother noted that some other members of the family had "blood problems," often after an infection or exposure to mothballs. A pedigree below shows the affected individuals of the family. See Figure 68. Biochemically, generation of which of the following cofactors is impaired in this patient?

A. $FADH_2$

B. NADH

C. NADPH

D. $FMNH_2$

E. Cobalamin

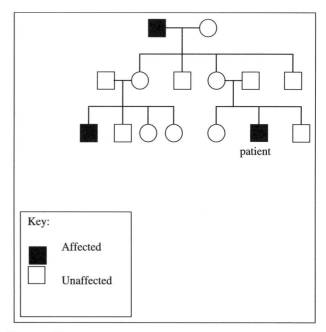

Figure 68

69. A 12-year-old male presents to your office with a complaint of having spells characterized by a vacant, staring expression and slight muscle twitching of the face. These episodes occur many times during the day and last for several seconds. Which of the following is the preferred maintenance drug for this child?

A. Phenytoin

B. Carbamazepine

C. Ethosuximide

D. Phenobarbital

E. Lamotrigine

70. A 55-year-old black male with a 40-year history of cigarette smoking is diagnosed with adenocarcinoma of the lung. Regardless of the initiating event, the lung cancer in the patient is dependent on the presence of multiple genetic alterations. Which of the following statements about the genetic changes involved in cancer development is most accurate?

A. Tumor suppressor genes and oncogenes undergo loss-of-function mutations.

B. Tumor suppressor genes and oncogenes undergo gain-of-function mutations.

C. Tumor suppressor genes undergo gain of function mutations and oncogenes undergo loss-of function mutations.

D. Tumor suppressor genes undergo loss of function mutations and oncogenes undergo gain of function mutations.

E. None of the above.

71. After an uneventful football practice, a 13-year-old junior high school athlete develops nausea, vomiting, neck pain, and headache at home. During the next hour, he's more tired and feels sedated. His mother brings him to the ER. As an intern, you find that he's febrile, has a weak pulse, and complains of pain on neck flexion and leg stretching. You perform a lumbar puncture. List the anatomical layers the needle would traverse from the outside to the inside to obtain the CSF fluid.

A. Skin, subcutaneous tissue, interspinous ligament, ligamentum flavum, supraspinous ligament, dura mater, arachnoid mater

B. Skin, subcutaneous tissue, supraspinous ligament, interspinous ligament, ligamentum flavum, dura mater, arachnoid mater

C. Skin, subcutaneous tissue, ligamentum flavum, supraspinous ligament, interspinous ligament, dura mater, arachnoid mater

D. Skin, supraspinous ligament, interspinous ligament, ligamentum flavum, dura mater, arachnoid mater, subcutaneous tissue

E. Skin, subcutaneous tissue, supraspinous ligament, interspinous ligament, ligamentum flavum, arachnoid mater, dura mater

72. During your neurology rotation your team is taking care of a 58-year-old man with a disorder that has resulted in several distressing symptoms. An MRI reveals marked atrophy of the frontal lobes. Which of the following would the man most likely be experiencing as a result of this abnormality?

A. Temperature dysregulation

B. Bitemporal hemianopia

C. Intention tremor

D. Normal concentration

E. Socially inappropriate comments

73. A 68-year-old female has been a patient in the hospital for 10 days. She was initially admitted for treatment of a community-acquired pneumonia. Over the last two days she has had diarrhea. On your morning rounds, you find that she has a high fever, continues to produce foul-smelling watery diarrhea, and has now become confused. What is the appropriate next step?

A. Sputum culture

B. Bronchoscopy

C. Skin test for TB

D. Stool culture

E. Stool assay for toxin

74. A 56-year-old man complains of two weeks of intermittent fevers and fatigue. He denies any upper respiratory symptoms and states that no one else in the household has been ill. When asked about his past medical history, he states that he has no problems except having been told that he had a heart murmur when he was 18. He also states that he has poor dentition and has had numerous root canals, the last one being about four weeks ago. The physical exam is significant for conjunctival petechiae bilaterally, splinter hemorrhages in the fingernail beds, and a III/VI systolic murmur heard best at the apex. CBC shows leukocytosis with a left shift, but other labs are normal. An echocardiogram is done and three sets of blood cultures are sent to the laboratory. What is the best empiric treatment?

A. No antibiotics at this time—wait for culture results
B. Nafcillin
C. Nafcillin and gentamicin
D. Vancomycin and gentamicin
E. Cefepime and gentamicin

75. An elderly woman is seen in the clinic with trembling hands, flat face, and slow speech. On physical exam, there is cogwheel rigidity of the wrists, postural instability, and dementia. What drug (legal or illegal) is associated with her condition?

A. Pyridium
B. Methimazole
C. 3,4-methylenedioxymethamphetamine (MDMA)
D. 1-methyl-4-phenyl-1,2,3,6- tetrahydropyridine (MPTP)

76. Renewal of which of the following antioxidants is dependent on the generation of a reduced niacin-derived cofactor by the hexose monophosphate shunt pathway?

A. Glutathione
B. Ascorbic acid
C. Tocopherol
D. Cholecalciferol
E. Retinoic acid

77. A 67-year-old man is brought to the emergency room immediately following a car accident. On examination, he is very anxious and breathing quickly. His blood pressure is 90/50 mm Hg, his heart rate is 130 beats per minute, his neck veins are collapsed, and his abdomen is tender. His lungs are clear to auscultation. His family tells you that he had a "minor heart attack" one month prior to the accident, but was otherwise healthy. A Swan-Ganz catheter reveals a pulmonary capillary wedge pressure (PCWP) of 1 mm Hg (normal 2 to 10 mm Hg) and decreased cardiac output. Based on the given information, which of the following types of shock most accurately characterizes this patient?

A. Cardiogenic shock
B. Neurogenic shock
C. Hypovolemic shock
D. Septic shock

78. A 65-year-old white male presents with atrial fibrillation. You decide to place him on long-term anticoagulation. The anticoagulant you choose inhibits vitamin K-dependent clotting factors. These factors are:

A. II, IV, VI, X
B. III, XII, IX, X
C. II, VII, IX, X
D. All of the above
E. None of the above

79. A 23-year-old man presents to the emergency department because his feet hurt after having walked the city streets for "seven days and seven nights gathering his army." As you are interviewing him he interrupts you several times to tell you that other people want to talk to him because he is, in fact, "a soldier of the lord" and everyone on the street knows him as "Knowledge." His speech is rapid and pressured. Urine drug screen and toxicology screen were negative. You make the diagnosis of bipolar disorder, acute mania. The lifetime risk of developing bipolar disorder is:

A. Up to 30%, with women affected twice as much as men
B. 10% in men and 5% in women
C. Equally common among men and women, about 1% in the general population, and up to 5 to 10% in first-degree relatives
D. Equally common among men and women, about 1% in the general population, with a greater prevalence among lower socio-economic groups, and 10 to 15% if a parent also is affected
E. Dependent on the degree and length of sun exposure received each day

80. A 65-year-old white man is returning for a follow-up appointment. He came to your office two weeks ago because of difficulty with urination. A digital prostate exam at that time was unremarkable. The PSA is 3.0. His BP on the initial visit was 145/105. Today his BP is similar. Which of the following drugs would you start?

A. A beta-blocker

B. An ACE inhibitor

C. An alpha-blocker

D. A diuretic

E. A calcium channel blocker

81. A 29-year-old woman who leads youth groups on hiking trips in northwestern New Jersey goes to her doctor with a red rash on her right calf. She says it has appeared in the last week, after a hiking trip two weeks ago, and has been growing in size. The doctor sends the patient's blood out for an ELISA test against *Borrelia burgdorferi* antibodies, to confirm his suspected diagnosis. If left untreated, which of these consequences is most likely to occur during the third, or late, stage of the suspected disease?

A. Bell's palsy

B. Myocarditis

C. Encephalopathy

D. Multiple, small erythema chronicum migrans

E. Transient musculoskeletal pain

82. During the age of wooden sailing vessels, sailors on long voyages were often plagued by bleeding gums, petechiae, and poor wound healing. Those symptoms vanished with the implementation of the practice of stocking ships' pantries with citrus fruits. In modern times, this condition is only seen in chronic alcoholics and in others with poor nutritional intake. Which of the following biochemical pathways in collagen synthesis is hindered in these individuals?

A. Recognition of the signal peptide sequence in the nascent polypeptide allowing insertion of the polypeptide into the rough endoplasmic reticulum

B. Cleavage of the signal peptide within the rough endoplasmic reticulum to yield the collagen pro-alpha-chain

C. Posttranslational hydroxylation of proline and lysine residues

D. Formation of interchain di-sulfide bonds between pro-alpha-chains

E. Extracellular cleavage of N- and C-terminal propeptides

83. A 23-year-old resting male who has a blood pressure of 126/84 and heart rate of 65 is given unknown drug A followed by drug B. After administration of drug A, the patient's blood pressure becomes 156/98 and has a heart rate of 66. Following administration of drug B, the patient's blood pressure becomes 118/78 and heart rate of 48. Based upon the patient information, what are the likely possibilities of drug A and B?

Drug A   Drug B

A. Phenylephrine Propranolol

B. Prazosin Metoprolol

C. Propranolol Dobutamine

D. Phentolamine Isoproteranol

84. A concerned African-American woman brings her 3-year-old to the clinic. She knows "not to give baby aspirin to babies." The child has had a "cold" and she has been using an over-the-counter decongestant and giving him children's Motrin. A CBC reveals him to be anemic and his red cells are not spherocytic. Clinical investigation points to hemolysis secondary to G6PD-deficiency. Which one of the following is the most likely cause of this episode?

A. Pseudoephedrine

B. Ibuprofen

C. Aspirin

D. Episode not related to medication

E. Tylenol

85. A 50-year-old female presents to her primary care physician's office 18 months after the death of her husband due to cancer. Since losing her husband, she has experienced a lack of interest in activities she previously enjoyed. She has also had a decreased appetite and she frequently suffers from insomnia. The patient states her energy level is poor and she feels fatigued all of the time. She expresses an inability to concentrate on simple daily activities. The physician notes that she is easily tearful and expresses feelings of sadness and hopelessness. The patient has no significant past medical history. Routine screening laboratory tests and physical exam are within normal limits. Which of the following is the most likely diagnosis for this patient?

A. Bereavement

B. Mood disorder due to medical illness

C. Dysthymic disorder

D. Major depressive disorder

E. Seasonal affective disorder

86. An 18-month-old boy is brought to his pediatrician by his parents. Mom states that her son has a rash all over his body. She states that her son did have a fever of 103 degrees for which she took him to the emergency room. He was given an antipyretic that did not help him. He has no coughing, sneezing, runny nose, or tugging on ears. Activity and appetite are normal. After three to four days mom noticed that the fever disappeared but a rash appeared on his belly. She did not think it was anything until the next day when the rash (maculopapular) spread all over his body. The best explanation for the above finding is:

    A. Paramyxovirus ss(–)RNA
    B. Herpes virus dsDNA enveloped
    C. Parvovirus B-19 ssDNA naked
    D. Human herpes virus 6 (HHV-6)
    E. Togavirus ss(+)RNA

87. During your first clinical rotation you encounter a 12-month-old child with hypotonia, microcephaly, a slanted appearance to the eyes, a large protruding tongue, and broad, short hands with a transverse palmar crease. He has a loud systolic heart murmur. The incidence of this condition is increased when the maternal age is:

    A. Above 35
    B. Under 35, over 20
    C. Under 20
    D. Cannot be determined based on the information given

88. A 45-year-old male alcoholic has been hospitalized for vomiting for the past seven days. Which of the following acid-base values would be expected in this patient?

    A. pH 7.88 / paO$_2$ 70 / paCO$_2$ 55 / HCO$_3$ 35
    B. pH 7.88 / paO$_2$ 90 / paCO$_2$ 40 / HCO$_3$ 35
    C. pH 7.44 / paO$_2$ 90 / paCO$_2$ 40 / HCO$_3$ 24
    D. pH 7.33 / paO$_2$ 60 / paCO$_2$ 60 / HCO$_3$ 25
    E. pH 7.33 / paO$_2$ 60 / paCO$_2$ 60 / HCO$_3$ 30

89. A 49-year-old alcoholic man is brought to the emergency room with nausea, vomiting, and abdominal pain. His friend states that the patient had been drinking "wood alcohol" (methanol). Methanol is metabolized by alcohol dehydrogenase to its toxic metabolite, formic acid. In addition to administering fluids and bicarbonates to increase renal clearance of formic acid, ethanol is administered. What is the mechanism of action of ethanol in the treatment of methanol overdose?

    A. Allosteric inhibition of alcohol dehydrogenase
    B. Shortening the half-life of methanol in the circulation
    C. Competitive inhibition of alcohol dehydrogenase
    D. Allosteric activation of alcohol dehydrogenase

90. An unconscious 45-year-old male is brought to the emergency room suffering from a hypertensive crisis and hyperthermia. The patient's wife states that her husband had recently been discharged from the hospital for treatment of atypical depression. Since his discharge, the wife states that her husband had been doing well, and just prior to being rushed to the emergency room, she and her husband had been enjoying themselves at a wine and cheese cocktail party. Which of the following medication was the patient most likely being treated with for his depression?

    A. Tranylcypromine
    B. Fluoxetine
    C. Amitriptyline
    D. Bupropion
    E. Clomipramine

91. A 35-year-old white male art metal worker has been cleaning metal with an unknown cleaner. He presents with giddiness, hyperpnea, and headache followed rapidly by cyanosis and unconsciousness. His breath has the odor of "bitter almonds." What is the appropriate treatment for his condition?

    A. Administration of dimercaprol
    B. Administration of protamine
    C. Administration of nitrite
    D. Administration of deferoxamine
    E. Administration of lidocaine

92. A 4-year-old white male child presents with honey crusted skin lesions of a few days duration on his face and hands. **See Figure 92.** If you were to culture the fluid when the crust is ruptured you would find:

    A. Gram-positive cocci in chains; catalase negative; beta-hemolytic; bacitracin-resistant
    B. dsDNA-linear enveloped; icosahedral; replicates in the nucleus
    C. Gram-positive cocci in chains; catalase negative; beta-hemolytic; bacitracin sensitive OR gram-positive cocci in clusters; catalase positive; beta-hemolytic; coagulase positive
    D. dsDNA-linear; enveloped; brick shaped; replicates in the cytoplasm

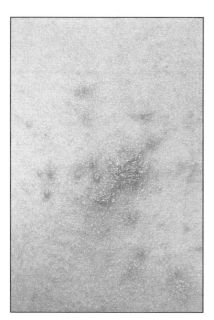

Figure 92 Reproduced with permission from Axford. Medicine. Blackwell Science, Ltd., 1996.

93. While on vacation in the Philippines, you come across a native Filipino man who is sitting on a bench wailing in pain. Being an inquisitive young doctor, you ask him to show you the problem. He promptly displays a swollen left foot. Upon closer inspection, the first metatarsal phalangeal joint is swollen, hot, and painful to touch. You quickly take him to the local doctor, who aspirates 10 cc of joint fluid. On microscopic examination, the fluid contains no bacteria and crystals that are free-floating and negatively birefringent.

    Which of the following would be the most likely diagnosis?

    A. CREST syndrome
    B. Pseudogout
    C. Gout
    D. Cellulitis
    E. Adenosine deaminase deficiency

94. A 36-year-old white female international aid worker living in the United States presents to your office with the onset of influenza-like symptoms, a cyclic fever, and generalized malaise that includes abdominal pain and profuse sweating. The patient has an extensive travel history in the African subcontinent. Also, the patient was diagnosed and treated 10 months ago for malaria with a single drug regimen while in Africa and with a prophylactic for three months after returning to the United States. The peripheral blood smear, as shown,

confirms the presence of trophozoites in the erythrocytic cycle. **See Figure 94.** The best pharmacological treatment for this patient is:

A. Quinine
B. Artesunate
C. Pyrimethamine and sulfadoxine
D. Amodiaquine and primaquine
E. Mefloquine

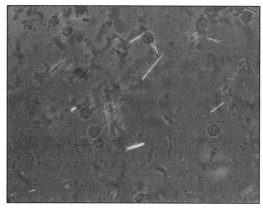

Figure 94 Reproduced with permission from Axford. Medicine. Blackwell Science, Ltd., 1996.

95. You are assisting with the delivery of a baby during your obstetrical rotation. A genotypically female patient is delivered with ambiguous genitalia, clitoral hypertrophy, and partial fusion of the labioscrotal folds. On the fourth day after delivery, the neonate's laboratory studies reveal severe hyponatremia, hyperkalemia, metabolic acidosis, and high levels of ACTH. Which enzyme deficiency in the adrenal steroidogenesis pathway accounts for this patient's condition?

    A. 11β-hydroxylase
    B. Aldosterone synthase
    C. 21β-hydroxylase
    D. 17β-dehydrogenase
    E. Lyase

96. Of the following diseases, which one usually causes death within the first year of life?

    A. Edward's syndrome
    B. Patau's syndrome
    C. Von Hippel-Lindau disease
    D. All of the above
    E. A and C only
    F. A and B only

97. You are observing a sleep study on one of your patients. His pulse, blood pressure, and respirations are all increased from his baseline. What kind of pattern would you see on an EEG during this stage?

   A. Alpha waves and low voltage activity

   B. Low voltage, sawtooth waves

   C. Delta waves and high voltage activity

   D. Sleep spindles and K complexes

   E. Theta waves, low voltage activity

98. Propranolol would be an appropriate choice of medication for which of the following patients?

   A. An elderly patient with long-standing glaucoma

   B. A female with frequent migraine headaches

   C. A male with coronary artery disease that presents with acute myocardial infarction

   D. A 60-year-old male with stable chronic angina

   E. All of the above

99. During a summer heat wave, a 33-year-old female landscaper is admitted to the hospital for intermittent, sharp, stabbing pain in her right flank that became progressively worse before coming to the hospital. On admission, the patient had a pulse of 110, blood pressure of 142/88, and respirations of 22. You begin treatment for dehydration and kidney stones. The next day, you review the patient's lab data and visit with her at the bedside. Her urine creatinine concentration is 120 mg/dL with a plasma creatinine concentration of 2.0 mg/dL. The 24-hour urine volume is 1440 ml. What is the creatinine clearance of this patient?

   A. 60 ml/min

   B. 120 ml/min

   C. 75 ml/min

   D. 40 ml/min

   E. 78 ml/min

100. A 25-year-old male construction worker is having difficulty raising his right shoulder, rotating his right scapula, and abducting and flexing his right arm. He says that he received a blow to his neck from a large beam. At what area of his neck did the trauma occur?

   A. Carotid triangle

   B. Posterior triangle

   C. Submandibular triangle

   D. Anterior triangle

BLOCK II - ANSWER KEY

51-E	64-C	77-C	89-C
52-D	65-E	78-C	90-A
53-D	66-E	79-C	91-C
54-E	67-E	80-C	92-C
55-E	68-C	81-C	93-C
56-C	69-C	82-C	94-D
57-C	70-D	83-A	95-C
58-E	71-B	84-B	96-F
59-D	72-A	85-D	97-B
60-E	73-E	86-D	98-E
61-E	74-C	87-A	99-A
62-E	75-D	88-A	100-B
63-C	76-A		

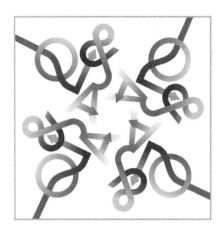

ANSWERS
BLOCK 2

51. E The arterial supply of the diaphragm consists of the phrenic arteries and the musculophrenic and pericardiophrenic arteries (latter two are branches of the internal thoracic artery).

A. 95% of diaphragmatic ruptures occur on the left due to the protection afforded on the right by the liver.
B. The celiac artery emerges after the aorta passes through the diaphragm and enters the abdomen.
C. Both phrenic nerves pass through the diaphragm and innervate the abdominal side.
D. The motor supply of the diaphragm (phrenic nerves) arises from the ventral roots of C3-C5.

52. D Developmental theorist Erik Erikson identified eight stages of psychological development from birth throughout one's life. In each stage, a major task confronts the individual and the manner in which the individual handles the task affects his/her future development. Generativity vs. self-absorption is the stage between ages 30 to 65 and involves either continued productivity or a sense of stagnation. Changes in work and relationships are common in this stage.

A. This is the stage associated with ages 6 to 12 years and involves success in school with the task of achieving competency in demands of school and society.
B. This stage is associated with age over 65 years and the task is having pride in accomplishments or worthlessness.

C. This stage takes place between ages 3 to 6 years when a child starts to take risks and become aware of potential punishment. If the task is met, the individual is more likely to become a responsible and self-disciplined adult.
E. This stage occurs between ages 1 to 3 years when the goal is to achieve a sense of autonomy separate from the parental figure.

53. D The brain cannot survive on any energy fuel other than glucose or ketones. It prefers glucose, but will use ketones under conditions of glucose deprivation. In a normal fasting individual, the brain derives its energy primarily from glycogenolysis in the first 24 hours. For the rest of the first week, the brain of the normal fasting individual will derive its energy primarily from gluconeogenesis, and this primarily from protein catabolism (using mostly the amino acid alanine from protein breakdown in muscle). To prevent excess protein breakdown, the brain then switches to ketogenesis as its primary source of energy, the ketones being derived from fatty acids. This switch occurs because as acetyl CoA accumulates in the brain (derived from ketone metabolism, which starts to occur during the first week of fasting, though is not predominant), pyruvate dehydrogenase (PDH) becomes inhibited by it, thereby slowing the metabolism of glucose and further favoring the metabolism of ketones. Though this is the normal sequence of events, our patient has a deficiency in a key enzyme of gluconeogenesis. Thus, the process of gluconeogenesis is compromised and ketogenesis would be the primary source of fuel for the brain after the first day.

54. E *M. tuberculosis* is best grown on Lowenstein-Jensen medium, which consists of egg yolk and malachite green to suppress growth of contaminants. Culturing the bacteria takes about six weeks.

A. The BCG vaccine is widely used in other parts of the world, including Mexico. It is used rarely if at all in this country.
B. A positive PPD test indicates the body has formed a secondary response to *M. tuberculosis* and has at one time encountered the pathogen. This does not indicate an ongoing infection.
C. TB is most commonly transmitted by air droplets.
D. The initial infection with *M. tuberculosis* is in the lower lobes of the lungs. If there is secondary TB this will typically occur in the apex of the lungs where there is little circulation and thus less immune response.

55. E This patient is suffering from Zollinger-Ellison syndrome. This condition is caused by a gastrinoma of the pancreas or the upper duodenum and is associated with gastrin hypersecretion and thus acid overproduction. Omeprazole is a direct inhibitor of the proton pump and is efficacious in Zollinger-Ellison syndrome.

A. Sucralfate polymerizes into a sticky gel that covers ulcers and inhibits further acidic damage. Sucralfate is a pro drug that requires a pH below 4.0. An antacid will prevent sucralfate from polymerizing.

B. Metoclopramide is a cholinomimetic agent and a D2 blocker. It is an antiemetic agent and a prokinetic agent, promoting gastrointestinal motility. It will not decrease acid production.

C. Fexofenadine is an antihistamine and an H1 blocker. It is used to relieve allergy symptoms, not decrease acid production.

D. Diphenoxylate is an antidiarrheal agent that decreases gastrointestinal peristalsis. It does not affect acid levels in the stomach.

56. C The aggressive nature of adenocarcinoma of the esophagus is due largely to the lack of a serosa in the esophagus.

A. The metaplasia is squamous to columnar in the precursor lesion, Barrett's esophagus.

B. Esophageal cancer, particularly squamous cell cancer, occurs far more frequently in patients who drink and/or smoke.

D. Long-standing reflux does lead to Barrett's esophagus.

E. Sliding esophageal hernias, obesity, and sphincter incompetence all lead to an increased risk of esophagitis.

57. C Idiopathic pulmonary fibrosis is a type of interstitial lung disease that is characterized clinically by exertional dyspnea, a nonproductive cough, and steadily deteriorating lung function. Chest radiograph reveals patchy, reticular, or ground glass opacities. Pulmonary function testing follows a restrictive pattern, characterized by decreased TLC and normal to increased FEV_1/FVC. The five-year survival rate following diagnosis of idiopathic pulmonary fibrosis is 30 to 50%.

A. Asthma is an obstructive lung disease, characterized by episodic wheezing responding to bronchodilators. Obstructive lung diseases are characterized by a decreased FEV_1/FVC ratio and normal to increased TLC.

B. Emphysema is an obstructive lung disease, characterized by a decreased FEV_1/FVC ratio and normal to increased TLC.

D. Chronic bronchitis is also an obstructive lung disease, characterized by wheezing, a productive cough, a decreased FEV_1/FVC ratio and normal to increased TLC.

58. E Mucor is classic in causing a rapid infection to the sinuses in immunocompromised patients, such as those in DKA, or those who are neutropenic. The amphotericin B should clue one in that a fungal infection is the cause.

A. *Staph aureus* would not be this rapid nor would amphotericin B be used in the treatment regimen.

B. *Pseudomonas aeurginosa* would not be treated with amphotericin B and would not be this rapid.

C. *Clostridium perfringens* would rarely be the culprit in a rapid infection in a patient who was hospitalized.

D. Although *Aspergillus* causes infection in immunocompromised patients, its progress is not as rapid as described and it classically presents as a lung infection.

59. D PCP does not typically produce tolerance or withdrawal symptoms. Tolerance is a phenomenon by which the body becomes increasingly resistant to the effects of a substance with continued exposure. Withdrawal produces physiological changes and symptoms that occur when some substances are withdrawn or markedly reduced after a period of prolonged use. Typical drugs to produce withdrawal symptoms include tranquilizers, narcotics, stimulants, barbiturates, and alcohol. Withdrawal may be life threatening, such as delirium tremens that occurs after alcohol withdrawal.

A. Nicotine is a substance that commonly results in tolerance and withdrawal.

B. Alcohol is a substance that commonly results in tolerance and withdrawal.

C. Caffeine is a substance that commonly results in tolerance and withdrawal.

E. Benzodiazepines are substances that commonly result in tolerance and withdrawal.

60. E The fever with unproductive cough associated with a chest x-ray demonstrating interstitial infiltrates indicates that this patient is suffering from an atypical pneumonia. The four main bacterial organisms responsible for atypical pneumonia are *Legionella pneumophila*, *Chlamydia pneumoniae*, *Coxiella burnetii*, and *Mycoplasma pneumoniae*. A "typical" pneumonia would be one associated with fever, chills, cough, sputum production, and lobar consolidation (the latter evidenced by bronchial breath sounds, egophony, increased tactile fremitus, and dullness to percussion). Some of the organisms associated with typical lobar pneumonia include *Streptococcus pneumoniae*, *Klebsiella pneumoniae*, *Haemophilus influenzae*, *Moraxella catarrhalis*, and *Mycobacteriae tuberculosis*. The main features of atypical pneumonia include a lack of sputum production as well as minor findings upon pulmonary exam. The chest x-ray commonly demonstrates interstitial infiltrates, at times more prominent than would be predicted by auscultation of the chest. The most common type of pneumonia (atypical or classic) found in adolescents and young adults is *Mycoplasma pneumoniae*. This organism is spread by close contact (such as is found within dormitories and military barracks), via respiratory droplets. In addition, the skin lesions described in the case are classic for erythema multiforme, common in infections caused by *Mycoplasma pneumoniae*. This skin lesion is not associated with any of the other pneumonia-causing organisms. Thus, one should initially assume that this patient is suffering from an atypical pneumonia caused by the bacteria *Mycoplasma pneumoniae*. This organism is a small extracellular bacteria that does not contain a cell wall (i.e., no peptidoglycan), and as such is not affected by penicillins or cephalosporins (among other antibiotics that inhibit cell wall synthesis), nor is it visible on Gram's stain. Although it contains a cell membrane full of sterols, it is unable to synthesize them itself. Thus, it must obtain cholesterol from its environment. Cold agglutinins present within the serum are found in 65% of *Mycoplasma pneumoniae* infections. Erythromycin, clarithromycin, and azithromycin are treatment options.

A. This is characteristic of *Chlamydia pneumoniae*, not *Mycoplasma pneumoniae*.

B. This is true of *Chlamydia pneumoniae* and *Coxiella burnetii*, but not *Mycoplasma pneumoniae*. *Legionella pneumophila* on the other hand is a facultative intracellular bacteria.

C. This is true of *Moraxella catarrhalis*, a cause of classic lobar pneumonia in elderly patients with chronic obstructive pulmonary disease (COPD).

D. This is true of *Legionella pneumophila*, the organism responsible for Legionnaire's disease (atypical pneumonia, mental confusion, and diarrhea), but not *Mycoplasma pneumoniae*, whose reservoir is the human respiratory tract itself.

61. E Flumazenil is a benzodiazepine receptor antagonist and is used to reverse the sedative effects of benzodiazepines.

A. The best therapy for lead toxicity is CaEDTA and dimercaprol. Penicillamine can be used but is not the best choice.

B. The appropriate therapy for streptokinase overdose is aminocaproic acid.

C. The appropriate reversal agent for opioids is naloxone, a competitive narcotic antagonist.

D. The appropriate treatment for warfarin overdose is vitamin K and FFP.

62. E The ureters are at a high risk of damage any time the uterine arteries are being operated on. At the level of the cervix, the ureters pass directly under the uterine arteries. **See Figure 62.** Before the uterine arteries are ligated, the ureters must be identified and protected.

A. The uterine arteries are branches of the internal thoracic artery.

B. The main blood supply of the uterus (uterine artery) travels in the broad ligament.

C. The broad ligament contains the blood supply to the uterus and uterine tubes. It does support the uterus, but that is not its primary function.

D. The ovarian arteries branch directly off of the aorta.

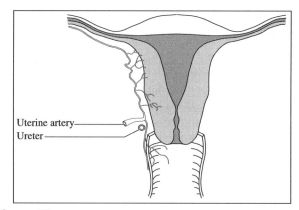

Figure 62

63. C This patient has ulcerative colitis. The lesions in ulcerative colitis extend from the rectum and continue uninterrupted, in contrast to Crohn's disease. Additionally, the ulcerations are superficial and do not extend to the serosa, causing fissuring, as in Crohn's. Surgical outcome for ulcerative colitis is generally curative.

A. Crohn's disease is characterized by transmural inflammatory involvement of the bowel with noncaseating granulomas and fissures exhibiting skipping phenomena. Because of the skip lesions, surgical prognosis is generally poor.

B. Incorrect. See A.

D. Neutrophilic infiltration of the muscularis is characteristic of appendicitis.

E. Small spherical outpouchings of atrophic mucosa with absent muscularis propria alongside the taenia coli is characteristic of diverticulosis.

64. C Vigorous exercise would result in a drop in pH and an increase in carbon dioxide, both of which would result in a right shift in the curve to facilitate higher oxygen delivery to peripheral tissues. Curve A is incorrect as this curve demonstrates the curve for fetal hemoglobin, as it has to have a higher oxygen affinity than maternal hemoglobin to deliver oxygen to the fetus.

Curve B would be expected in someone who was alkalotic or had a decreased amount of carbon dioxide in their body, i.e., someone who was hyperventilating.

65. E Metronidazole has a disulfiram (Antabuse) reaction when combined with alcohol. The patient is unable to metabolize alcohol properly and becomes violently ill.

A. Although tetracycline can alter liver enzymes, it is unlikely to alter them to the point that such a comparatively small amount of alcohol could cause liver dysfunction.

B. Propranolol has no specific toxic interaction with alcohol.

C. Buspirone has no specific toxic interaction with alcohol.

D. Diphenhydramine would cause a greater sedation effect when combined with alcohol as compared to becoming violently ill.

66. E Stranger anxiety is a normal stage of development occurring generally between 7 to 9 months of age. Of the milestones listed, the infant's ability to recognize strangers would be the most "advanced."

A. Cooing generally occurs by 3 months.

B. The ability to bring hands to midline generally occurs at 4 months.

C. Social smile occurs around 2 months.

D. The ability to hold head up steadily generally occurs at 3 months.

67. E Bladder carcinoma is frequently seen in Egypt as a consequence of chronic infection with *Schistosoma haematobium*. The ova of this organism (unlike the two discussed in answer D) invade through the bladder wall as a part of its life cycle. Praziquantel or metrifonate may be used against *S. haematobium*.

A. Chronic *E. coli* urinary tract infections are not associated with bladder carcinoma.

B. Acute urinary tract infections with *E. coli* are not associated with bladder carcinoma.

C. Infection with adenovirus serotype 11 can cause acute hemorrhagic cystitis, in which hematuria and dysuria are prominent clinical findings, but is not associated with bladder carcinoma.

D. *Schistosoma mansoni* and *S. japonicum* are blood fluke infections, but do not involve the bladder (as does *S. haematobium*). Instead, their life cycle involves invasion through the bowel mucosa, which can lead to congestion, thickening, and ulceration of the bowel. Eggs deposited in the large intestine may lead to periportal fibrosis and hepatomegaly if they lodge in the presinusoidal capillaries as they are carried by portal blood back towards the liver.

68. C Glucose-6-phoshate dehydrogenase deficiency is an inherited metabolic disorder that usually does not become symptomatic until a stressor, such as infection, some medications such as ibuprofen, or certain foods (e.g., fava beans), or exposure to certain chemicals befalls the patient. The disorder is X-linked recessive, as strongly suggested by the family tree which shows only males among the affected. The biochemical pathway involved generates a reduced cofactor species, NADPH.

A. $FADH_2$ is generated by the electron transport system.

B. The pathway enzymes are specific for NADPH generation, not NADH.

D. $FMNH_2$ is involved in cytochrome P450 reductase and nitric oxide synthetase activity.

E. Cobalamin is involved in only two reactions, synthesis of methionine from homocysteine and conversion of methylmalonyl-CoA to succinyl CoA.

69. C This patient is experiencing absence seizures (also called petit mal). The onset of this disorder is often associated with puberty. With a seizure, the patient ceases all voluntary motor activity, assumes a vacant expression, and may or may not have some mild myoclonic activity. With the resumption of consciousness, the patient may resume speaking at exactly the point at which he left off. There is usually no aura or warning. Ethosuximide is the drug of choice in patients with absence seizures.

A. Phenytoin is not an effective treatment for patients with absence seizures.
B. Carbamazepine is not an effective treatment for patients with absence seizures.
D. Phenobarbital is not an effective treatment for patients with absence seizures.
E. Lamotrigine is not generally used to treat absence seizures. Also, the use of lamotrigine in children with epilepsy has not been studied.

70. D Tumor suppressor genes actively prevent genetic alterations. For example, *TP53* has been called the "guardian of the genome," for its role in initiating cell cycle arrest or apoptosis after DNA damage occurs. Loss of the protective function of these tumor suppressor genes contributes to carcinogenesis. Oncogenes, or proto-oncogenes as they are called before they mutate, serve normal growth-promoting functions that can be switched off if there is no more need for growth. They contribute to cancer development only after mutations result in protein products that can no longer be switched off. These oncogenes undergo a gain-of-function mutation.

A, B, C, and E are incorrect. See explanation above.

71. B The above patient has symptoms typical of meningitis. Lumbar puncture (spinal tap) is an important tool in diagnosing whether the cause is bacterial or viral. It is essential to know the different tissue layers that one would encounter when performing a lumbar puncture. They are skin, subcutaneous tissue, supraspinous ligament, interspinous ligament, ligamentum flavum, dura mater, arachnoid mater.

A. After the skin and the subcutaneous tissue, the supraspinous ligament is the next layer as it connects the apices of the spinous process from C7 to the sacrum.
C. Ligamentum flavum is encountered after the supraspinous ligament and the interspinous ligament. Ligamentum flavum (yellow ligament) joins the laminae of adjacent vertebral arches.

D. Subcutaneous tissue would be encountered after penetrating the skin.
E. The needle would encounter the dura mater and then the arachnoid layer. The arachnoid layer is not attached to the dura mater and is held against the inner surface of the dura mater by pressure of the CSF.

72. A The frontal lobes have multiple important functions and are primarily associated with "executive functioning," which includes mood regulation, orientation, concentration, and judging social situations and appropriate behaviors.

A. The hypothalamus controls temperature regulation.
B. This symptom is a result of damage or impingement to the optic chiasm.
C. Intention tremor would most likely be due to cerebellar dysfunction.
D. Concentration would likely be impaired.

73. E Stool assay for *Clostridium difficile* toxin is the correct answer. This patient has been treated with antibiotics for her pneumonia, which have resulted in an overgrowth of *Clostridium difficile*. Prompt diagnosis and treatment of *C. difficile* overgrowth with oral metronidazole or oral vancomycin may prevent development of pseudomembranous colitis and obviate the need for colectomy. In this patient with severe symptomatology (fever, mental status changes), flexible sigmoidoscopy may be performed to provide an even more rapid diagnosis so that treatment can be started.

A. Sputum culture is not likely to shed any light upon this patient's problem, which is now gastrointestinal.
B. Bronchoscopy is not likely to aid in diagnosis or treatment and will waste valuable time.
C. Placement of a TB skin test is not the correct answer. The patient's problem is antibiotic-induced diarrhea, which may be due to *C. difficile* overgrowth.
D. A stool culture may provide the diagnosis eventually, assuming that the lab is informed that *C. difficile* overgrowth is suspected. However, the most appropriate test is an assay for *C. difficile* toxin, since this will provide the desired information more quickly.

74. C A patient with this presentation of infective endocarditis probably has a gram-positive infection with *S. viridans*, as a complication of his dental work. For suspected gram-positive infective endocarditis, the empiric treatment is a penicillinase-resistant penicillin (nafcillin) and an aminoglycoside (gentamicin). This takes advantage of synergy where one antibiotic disrupts the cell wall and allows easier access for the second to do its work. Since endocarditis is often difficult to treat, synergy is important for a successful outcome.

A. Antibiotic treatment must be started because blood culture results will take too long. Infective endocarditis is a potentially fatal disease if left untreated.

B. Although nafcillin alone is effective against gram-positive infections, endocarditis infections are very difficult to eradicate, and a synergistic combination is preferred.

D. Vancomycin should be reserved for cases where nafcillin fails or for methicillin-resistant *S. aureus* infections.

E. Cefepime is used primarily for *Pseudomonas* infections. In this patient, gram-negative infective endocarditis is less likely.

75. D Parkinson's disease is a neurodegenerative disorder of the extrapyramidal system characterized by resting tremor, cogwheel rigidity, and bradykinesia. The pathology includes the loss of dopaminergic neurons in the substantia nigra and often is associated with Lewy bodies. 1-Methyl-4-phenyl-1,2,3,6-tetrahydropyridine (MPTP) is an illicit drug, formed from impure preparation of Demerol, that is associated with Parkinson's disease.

A. Pyridium (phenazopyridine) is an analgesic for urinary tract irritation.

B. Methimazole inhibits synthesis of thyroid hormones.

C. 3,4-methylenedioxymethamphetamine (MDMA or "ecstasy") is not associated with Parkinson's disease.

76. A Glucose-6-phosphate dehydrogenase (G6PD) generates NADPH, which in turn is utilized by glutathione reductase to produce reduced glutathione. It is reduced glutathione that is predominantly responsible for scavenging hydrogen peroxide in the cytoplasm of red blood cells. Individuals with G6PD deficiency may suffer hemolysis secondary to stress as reduced glutathione is not available to scavenge hydrogen peroxide, with cell membrane damage and hemolysis resulting.

B. Ascorbic acid (vitamin C) is an essential nutrient that must be obtained from the diet. Severe lack of ascorbic acid results in scurvy.

C. Tocopherol (vitamin E) is a fat-soluble essential nutrient.

D. Cholecalciferol (vitamin D) is a dietary requirement for those who do not receive sufficient sunlight exposure. Cholecalciferol is converted to biologically active forms, which are used for serum calcium regulation.

E. Retinoic acid (vitamin A) is a nutrient necessary for night vision.

77. C This patient is clearly presenting with shock, characterized by hypotension, tachycardia, tachypnea, and mental status changes. Hypovolemic shock occurs following acute blood loss and, similar to cardiogenic shock, is characterized by a decreased cardiac output. Hypovolemic shock is differentiated from cardiogenic shock by the absence of jugular venous distension, absence of pulmonary edema, and a decreased PCWP.

A. Patients with cardiogenic shock present with jugular venous distention, rales, and often an S3 gallop. Patients in cardiogenic shock have an increased PCWP.

B. Neurogenic shock, which may follow obvious head or spinal cord injury, usually leads to the finding of warm extremities, in contrast to the cool extremities in patients with hypovolemic or cardiogenic shock.

D. Septic shock is characterized by increased cardiac output and would be unlikely to immediately follow a car accident.

78. C Coumadin (warfarin) is the long-term anticoagulant of choice. The vitamin-K dependent factors are II, VII, IX, and X.

A, B, D, E are all incorrect.

79. C Bipolar illness is equally common among men and women, affecting about 1% in the general population, and up to 5 to 10% in first-degree relatives. There are no sharp distinctions based on socioeconomic status.

A. These statistics apply to unipolar major depression.

B. See above.

D. These statistics apply to schizophrenia.

E. See above.

80. C In this case, by using an alpha-blocker, we get a "two-for-one" deal. The alpha-blocker will work against both the hypertension and benign prostatic hypertrophy (BPH). It will relieve symptoms by reducing smooth muscle tone and vasodilation. Another medical treatment of BPH is finasteride, a 5-alpha-1-reductase inhibitor, blocking the conversion of testosterone to dihydrotestosterone (DHT).

A. Beta-blockers may help the hypertension, but not the BPH.
B. ACE inhibitors also will not help with BPH.
D. Diuretics are best used for patients with hypertension and congestive heart failure.
E. Calcium channel blockers slow down the heart and cause vasodilation. They are used to prevent ischemic cardiac disease.

81. C This patient is most likely suffering from Lyme disease, considering her exposure to wilderness areas in the Northeast and the presence of a rash on her leg. The presence of *Borrelia* antibodies will confirm the diagnosis. Encephalopathy is a sequelae of Lyme disease that most often occurs during the third, or late, stage of the disease. The encephalopathy is subacute and can affect memory, mood, sleep, and even language. The current treatment for Lyme disease is doxycycline.

A. Bell's palsy is a well-known occurrence during stage 2 of Lyme disease, characterized by paralysis of one side of the face.
B. Myocarditis or heart block occurs in about 10% of patients during stage 2. Heart block is usually AV nodal block. These symptoms usually resolve within weeks.
D. These rashes are similar to the one seen in stage 1—a red, flat rash that grows out. They are, however, smaller and more widely disseminated, and occur in the second stage.
E. Joint and muscle pain that is migratory in nature can occur, usually about six months after the original infection. It can affect the joints, tendons, and bursae, but usually there is an absence of swelling. In the third stage, there is arthritis, pain, and swelling limited to the joints.

82. C Scurvy, which is the condition described here, is due to inadequate vitamin C (ascorbic acid) intake. Vitamin C is a necessary cofactor for the posttranslational hydroxylation of proline and lysine residues. Failure of these reactions results in poorly formed collagen fibrils, resulting in fragile tissues that tend to separate and bleed.

A. This reaction is vitamin C-independent.
B. This reaction is dependent on a correct signal peptide. Mutations of this peptide will result in failure to direct peptide into the RER, with failure to secrete protein out of the cell.
D. Interchain di-sulfide bond formation is spontaneous, if all prior assembly steps have proceeded appropriately.
E. Inherited N- and C-propeptidase defects will not produce scurvy, but may manifest as Ehlers-Danlos syndrome, also known as "rubber man's disease."

83. A Phenylephrine is an alpha agonist that would result in peripheral vasoconstriction and an increase in blood pressure with no significant change in heart rate. Propranolol is a beta antagonist which would explain the following decrease in blood pressure because of its effects at α-2 receptors and a decrease in heart rate because of its effects on α-1 receptors.

B. Prazosin is an alpha antagonist and would result in a decrease in peripheral blood pressure even though metoprolol would have similar effects as seen with propranolol as both are beta antagonists.
C. Propranolol would not result in higher blood pressures and dobutamine would not result in lower blood pressures. However, if drug A were dobutamine and drug B was propranolol, this clinical scenario would be correct.
D. Phentolamine is an α-1 antagonist and would result in peripheral vasodilation and isoproterenol is an α-1 and α-2 agonist and would result in a higher blood pressure and heart rate.

84. B Several medications can cause hemolysis in G6PD-deficient patients. These are aspirin, INH, sulfa drugs, ibuprofen, and primaquine. Since the mother knows not to give aspirin (not for G6PD reason, but other reasons), and the two other drugs, pseudoephedrine and Tylenol (acetaminophen), do not cause hemolysis, by process of elimination, the answer is ibuprofen (Motrin).

A. This drug does not cause hemolysis in G6PD-deficient patients.
C. Mother has not given the patient aspirin.
D. The answers "none of the above" or "can't answer" or "not related to medication" rarely are the correct answers, and are definitely not in this case.
E. Tylenol is safe for G6PD-deficient patients.

85. D This patient displays signs and symptoms of major depressive disorder. Five or more of the following must be present for at least two weeks for a diagnosis of major depressive disorder: depressed mood, more often than not (required for diagnosis); decreased interest or pleasure in activities (required for diagnosis); changes in sleep, such as insomnia or hypersomnia; feelings of guilt or worthlessness; decreased ability to concentrate; changes in appetite; psychomotor changes, such as agitation or retardation; and suicidal thoughts.

A. Although bereavement follows a severe loss and can produce a depressive syndrome, the symptoms typically improve and disappear weeks to months after the precipitating event. Bereavement that does not resolve can evolve into major depressive disorder, as in this patient.

B. This patient is an otherwise healthy 50-year-old woman with no significant past medical history and a normal exam. A precipitating event for this patient's depression can also be identified.

C. Dysthymic disorder is a mild and chronic form of major depression in which symptoms are present for more than two years.

E. Seasonal affective disorder is similar to major depressive disorder, but it occurs in a seasonal pattern. It often arises in fall or winter and improves in spring or summer.

86. D Roseola infantum or exanthem subitum caused by HHV-6 (human herpes virus 6). It is preceded by a high fever without affecting the child's activity or appetite. After the fever leaves a macular/maculopapular rash appears in one area and spreads all over the body lasting for about 24 hours.

A. Rubeola (measles) is caused by a *Paramyxovirus*, ss(–)RNA, where the child presents with fever, cough, coryza, and conjunctivitis with photophobia.

B. Chicken pox or varicella, a dsDNA enveloped virus, presents with pruritic vesicles that break and crust over, spreading in a centripetal fashion.

C. Fifth disease is due to the Parvovirus B-19, ssDNA naked. Erythema of the cheeks gives the classic "slapped cheeks" appearance.

E. Rubella is a togavirus, ss(+)RNA. It presents with suboccipital lymphadenopathy. A maculopapular rash begins on the face and spreads everywhere.

87. A This child has Down syndrome. The risk of Down syndrome increases dramatically for pregnant women over the age of 35, and may be as high as 1 in 80 for women who are over 40. In most cases, particularly in the "elderly" mother, it arises as a chromosomal aberration caused by nondisjunction during cell division, resulting in an extra chromosome (21) in the G group. A much smaller number of cases are caused by translocation of chromosome 14 or 15 in the D group and chromosome 21 or 22. These translocations can occur at any maternal age, and the mother or father may be carriers for the translocation. The parents should have chromosomal analysis on themselves and be advised about the possibility of Down syndrome in future offspring.

B, C, D, see above.

88. A This patient will likely be experiencing metabolic alkalosis with compensatory respiratory acidosis. The vomiting will explain the loss of HCl and an accumulation of bicarbonate that would result in a higher pH. The bodily compensation to retain CO_2 would result in respiratory acidosis to compensate. As a result, answer A is the most correct choice.

B. It shows only primary metabolic alkalosis evident by the higher pH and the high bicarbonate concentration. However, the arterial oxygen and carbon dioxide concentrations are within normal limits, suggesting this is only primary alkalosis with no compensatory acidosis.

C. It reflects the values of a normal person.

D. This is a person who is acidotic. However, this acidosis is due to primary respiratory acidosis, i.e., someone who is extremely hypoxic, since there is no change in bicarbonate to compensate.

E. This, too, is a person who is acidotic due to primary respiratory acidosis, but also has some compensatory secondary metabolic alkalosis evidenced by the higher bicarbonate concentration.

89. C Ethanol works by competitive inhibition of alcohol dehydrogenase. By competing with methanol at the active site of alcohol dehydrogenase, the conversion of methanol to formaldehyde and formic acid is decreased. This is logical, since ethanol and methanol have similar structures.

A. Ethanol acts at the active site, not an allosteric site.

B. Ethanol increases the half-life of methanol in the circulation from 30 hours to 60 hours.

D. Ethanol acts at the active site, not an allosteric site.

90. A Tranylcypromine (Parnate) belongs to the monoamine oxidase (MAO) inhibitor class of antidepressants used to treat atypical depression (depression with psychosis). MAO inhibitors, when ingested with tyramine-containing foods such as aged cheese, alcohol, and yeast, can lead to elevated blood pressure, hypertensive crisis, headache, neck stiffness, sweating, nausea, vomiting, and visual problems. The most serious consequences are stroke and possibly death. Hypertensive crisis is a medical emergency with cerebral vascular accidents being one of the greatest concerns.

B. Fluoxetine (Prozac) belongs to the serotonin selective reuptake inhibitor (SSRI) class of antidepressants. Side effects most likely to occur include agitation, insomnia, and sexual dysfunction. SSRIs are also used to treat obsessive-compulsive disorder in addition to depression.

C. Amitriptyline (Elavil) belongs to the tricyclic class of antidepressants. Side effects include sedation, orthostatic hypotension, cardiac arrhythmias, and anticholinergic symptoms (dry mouth, urinary retention, constipation).

D. Bupropion (Wellbutrin, Zyban) belongs to the heterocyclic class of antidepressants. Side effects include insomnia, tachycardia, and agitation but the drug has fewer adverse sexual effects than some of the others. Also used for smoking cessation.

E. Clomipramine (Anafranil) belongs to the tricyclic class of antidepressants. Side effects include sedation, orthostatic hypotension, cardiac arrhythmias, and anticholinergic symptoms (dry mouth, urinary retention, constipation). Clomipramine is also used to treat obsessive-compulsive disorder.

91. C This patient is suffering from cyanide poisoning. Hydrocyanic acid or cyanide salts are used as cleaning agents for metal, and in research. It is naturally present in apricot seeds and there are a number of reported cases of children becoming poisoned by eating apricot seeds. The breath odor is pathognomonic. Treatment must begin immediately, with amyl nitrite by inhalation until sodium nitrite can be given intravenously. Cyanide reacts with iron in the ferric (+++) state only. It reacts with the trivalent iron of cytochrome oxidase and with methemoglobin to form cyanmethemoglobin. The result is an inhibition of intracellular respiration. The nitrite produces a high concentration of methemoglobin (HB-Fe+++) that drives the cyanide from the cytochrome oxidase to the methemoglobin. Thiosulfate is then administered to the patient, forming thiocyanate, which is relatively nontoxic and readily excreted in the urine.

A. Dimercaprol is used to treat lead poisoning.

B. Protamine is used to counteract heparin.

D. Deferoxamine is used to treat iron poisoning.

E. Lidocaine is used to treat ventricular tachycardia and is used as a local anesthetic.

92. C Impetigo is usually caused by *Strep pyogenes*, a gram-positive cocci in chains, catalase negative, beta hemolytic and bacitracin sensitive. There are occasions, however, when *Staph aureus* is causative. *Staph aureus* often causes a more extensive illness, such as scalded skin syndrome.

A. This is *Strep agalactiae*. It does not cause any dermatological infections. However it can cause neonatal meningitis when the newborn travels through the birth canal that can be colonized with this organism.

B. This is the varicella virus that causes chicken pox in children and not impetigo. The lesions start with a red-based, clear vesicle containing clear fluid. They are usually scattered and may be present over the entire body.

D. Variola virus causes smallpox. This particular virus has been eradicated since the late 1970s but is a possible biological weapon.

93. C Gout is an arthritis associated with crystal deposition due to either increased production (from an increase in the activity of xanthine oxidase) or decreased excretion of uric acid. The disease has a curious predilection for Pacific Islanders and men older than 30. In an acute gouty flair, the main principle of treatment is to use NSAIDs and wait to lower the uric acid later since rapid decreases can elicit another acute gouty attack.

A. CREST syndrome, or limited scleroderma, is a constellation of symptoms including calcinosis, Raynaud's phenomenon, esophageal dysmotility, sclerodactyly, and telangiectasia.

B. Pseudogout is similar in its presentation to gout but the main difference is the deposition of calcium pyrophosphate crystals, not uric acid.

D. Although cellulitis or septic arthritis can be mistaken for gout, especially in the acute setting, this patient's joint aspiration contains no bacteria and negatively birefringent crystals.

E. Adenosine deaminase deficiency causes severe combined immunodeficiency. SCID is an abnormality associated with T-cell and B-cell dysfunction and death typically by age 3.

94. D *Plasmodium vivax* malaria is the most prevalent type of malarial infection and is characterized by tertian (2 days, 48 hours) cycles of fever often accompanied with hepatosplenomegaly, anemia, headaches, and lethargy. The malarial parasite is a single-cell protozoan (plasmodium) of which only four types are capable of infecting humans from the bite of a female anopheles mosquito: *P. malariae, P. ovale, P. vivax, P. falciparum*. Of these four, only *P. ovale* and *P. vivax* can produce the dormant hypnozoite after the sporozoites invade liver parenchymal cells during the exoerythrocytic cycle. If not treated properly, symptoms will subside for several weeks or months and recur due to the latent liver form of the parasite. The drug primaquine is the only proven antimalarial agent effective against the liver (exoerythrocytic) forms of the malarial parasite. It is a tissue schizonticide and gametocide but is relatively ineffective against the asexual erythrocytic forms and therefore must be used in conjunction with an aminoquinoline derivative, such as chloroquine or amodiaquine.

A. Quinidine is an alkaloid that is effective against *P. falciparum* in nonsensitive (chloroquine resistant) areas but has no exoerythrocytic effectiveness. It has a toxic state side effect called cinchonism.

B. Artesunate is not effective against dormant hypnozoites. It is a cheaper antimalarial used most often in children infected with *P. falciparum* in a nonsensitive area.

C. Pyrimethamine and sulfadoxine are not effective against the dormant hypnozoite. It is an antimalarial drug combination that causes a synergistic sequential blockade of the parasite's ability to produce folic acid.

E. Mefloquine, an antimalarial drug, is ineffective against the liver stage of vivax malaria and causes flashbacks as a common CNS side effect.

95. C Progesterone and 17-hydroxyprogesterone are converted into 11-deoxycorticosterone and 11-deoxycortisol, respectively, via the enzyme 21-hydroxylase (CYP21A2). 21β-hydroxylase is found only in the zona glomerulosa and zona fasiculata of the adrenal gland. 21β-hydroxylase deficiency, usually an autosomal recessive disorder, is the most common cause of congenital adrenal hyperplasia (CAH), accounting for 90% of the cases. The shift of steroidogenesis into other pathways causes excess production of androgenic cortisol precursors. With this deficiency, the effects impact primarily sexual development, as well as mineralocorticoid and glucocorticoid balance. If not treated, hyponatremia, hyperkalemia, hypotension, salt wasting, and acidosis precede death.

A. This has a milder effect since 11-deoxycorticosterone can perform the same function, albeit weaker, as aldosterone in the absence of 11β-hydroxylase.

B. This is needed for the conversion of corticosterone into mineralocorticoids, like aldosterone, and its absence would not account for virilization.

D. 17β-dehydrogenase deficiency would obstruct the production of testosterone from androgens but not account for the hemodynamic and electrolyte imbalance.

E. Lyase is needed to convert 17β-hydroxypregnenolone and 17-hydroxyprogesterone into androgens.

96. F Edward's syndrome and Patau's syndrome both cause death within the first year of life.

A. Edward's syndrome is caused by trisomy 18. The incidence is 1 in 8000 live births. Rocker bottom feet and low-set ears and micrognathia are common signs but by no means pathognomonic.

B. Patau's syndrome is caused by trisomy 13. The incidence is 1 in 5000. Signs and symptoms include mental retardation, microcephaly, polydactyly, and congenital heart disease.

C. Von Hippel-Lindau disease is an autosomal dominant disease with findings of hemangioblastomas of the retina, cerebellum, and medulla. Many affected children later develop bilateral renal cell carcinoma, among other tumors.

D, E. See above.

97. B The patient is experiencing REM (rapid eye movement) sleep. This is characterized by an increase in pulse, respiration, and blood pressure. Dreams occur during REM sleep and there is near total paralysis of skeletal muscles. Low voltage, sawtooth waves are characteristic EEG findings in REM sleep.

A. This is the characteristic of EEGs when awake.

C. This is the appearance of an EEG during Stages 3 and 4 of sleep.

D. This is the appearance of a Stage 2 EEG.

E. This is the appearance of a Stage 1 EEG.

98. E Beta blockers are indicated for chronic glaucoma, the prophylactic treatment of migraines, after myocardial infarctions and in stable angina. They are also useful in hyperthyroidism. Nonselective beta blockers such as propranolol should not be used in restrictive lung diseases because they can cause bronchoconstriction and extreme asphyxiation.

A. Propranolol decreases intraocular pressure and is useful in treating chronic glaucoma.
B. Propranolol is indicated for the prophylactic treatment of migraines.
C. The use of propranolol after myocardial infarctions can lead to reduced infarct size and lessen the chance of dangerous arrhythmias afterwards.
D. Propranolol decreases cardiac oxygen requirement and can improve exercise tolerance in patients with angina.

99. A

Creatinine clearance (ml/min) =

$$\frac{[Creatinine]_{urine}(mg/dL)}{[Creatinine]_{plasma}(mg/dL)} \times urine\ flow\ rate\ (ml/min)$$

Remember: [U]/[PEE] times HOW MUCH YOU PEE

Or clinical equation used for estimation:

$$Cl_{cr} = \frac{(140 - Age) \times weight\ (kg)}{72 \times [Creatinine]_{plasma}} \times 0.85_{females\ only}$$

{the Cockroft-Gault Equation}

  Creatinine clearance is a measure of glomerular filtration rate (GFR), which is the volume of fluid filtered by the glomeruli per minute. Creatinine, a catabolic by-product of creatine phosphate, is filtered but not secreted nor absorbed. It is a sensitive indicator of renal function. Creatinine clearance normally is between 80 and 125 ml/min. Elevation of serum creatinine and BUN is called azotemia. Generally a ratio of BUN to creatinine of greater than 20:1 indicates an extrarenal cause of kidney dysfunction, although the ratio may be less in patients with underlying renal failure. Ratios less than 20:1 suggest a problem intrinsic to the kidneys. The most important aspect of creatinine clearance calculations is to know the exact time it takes to form the urine sample and the exact amount of creatinine present. If the kidneys are damaged by some disease process, the creatinine clearance will decrease and the serum creatinine concentration will increase. "Plugging and chugging" the values from the problem produces a result of 60 ml/min. Make sure you convert 24 hours into minutes.

100. B The posterior triangle contains CN XI (accessory nerve). **See Figure 100.** The accessory nerve provides innervation to the trapezius muscle, which is involved in raising the shoulder, rotating the scapula, and abducting and flexing the arm. It also provides innervation to the sternocleidomastoid muscle. A branch that does not go into the posterior triangle provides innervation to the soft palate and pharyngeal muscles.

A. The carotid triangle contains the external carotid artery and the laryngeal nerve.
C. The submandibular triangle contains CN XII (hypoglossal).
D. The anterior triangle contains no cranial nerve structures.

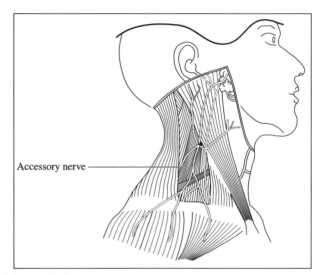

Accessory nerve

Figure 100

B, C, D, and **E** are incorrect.

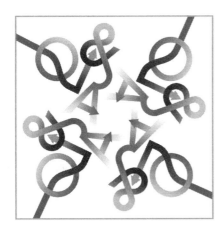

QUESTIONS
BLOCK 3

101. What is the disease caused by virulent proteins that intervene in the folding of normal proteins?

A. Progressive multifocal leukoencephalopathy

B. Kuru

C. Rabies

D. Measles

E. Dengue

102. A 42-year-old white female patient presents to your office with long-standing rheumatoid arthritis. She has been receiving ibuprofen 800 mg three times a day for one year and been on 40 mg of prednisone per day for approximately six weeks. In this patient, what side effects of these two drugs should you be most concerned about?

A. Weight loss

B. Hyperkalemia

C. Hypocalcemia

D. Liver toxicity

E. Anemia

103. A 47-year-old male has his right hand and arm caught in a trash compactor. Multiple fractures are seen on radiograph. The hand appears neurovascularly intact. Which bone, if fractured, is most likely to develop avascular necrosis (AVN)?

A. Midshaft radius

B. Midshaft ulna

C. Lunate

D. First metacarpal

E. Scaphoid

104. A 24-year-old Caucasian male presents to your office after having been on a regimen of isoniazid and rifampin for tuberculosis for three weeks. Yesterday he experienced the sudden onset of severe midepigastric abdominal pain, which has since been getting progressively worse, not relieved by aspirin or Tylenol. Associated with this have been episodes of nausea and vomiting. He also reports a dark color to his urine for the past week or so. His wife admits that he "had not been himself" for the past week or two, being very anxious, agitated, and even paranoid at times. Because of this, he had been taking a barbiturate for the past three days, the source of which they refuse to reveal. Heart rate is 110, blood pressure 145/85, respirations 24, temperature 99°F. While considering your differential diagnosis, you would want to rule out a rare deficiency in which of the following enzymes?

A. Cystathionine synthase

B. Homocysteine methyl transferase

C. Uroporphyrinogen synthase

D. Homogentisate oxidase

E. Branched-chain ketoacid dehydrogenase

F. Methylmalonyl-CoA mutase

105. A 22-year-old woman with a history of severe asthma presents to the emergency room with shortness of breath. Physical examination reveals prominent, diffuse, expiratory wheezing. She has minimal response to bronchodilators. On presentation, her arterial pCO_2 = 20 mm Hg. Over the next hour, she continues to have difficulty breathing, and her arterial pCO_2 increases to 40 mm Hg. On repeat physical examination, wheezing is decreased but she continues to be very uncomfortable and displays prominent use of accessory muscles of respiration. Which of the following is true about this patient?

A. The normalization of the patient's CO_2 level is reassuring.

B. Decreased wheezing is a reliable indicator of improved respiratory status.

C. Steroids will produce an immediate, dramatic improvement in respiratory status.

D. The patient's respiratory status is deteriorating.

106. A 15-year-old white female is brought to your office by her concerned mother who states that her daughter has been eating less and less and has been losing weight for the last 10 months. She weighs herself at least six times a day and has been found doing jumping jacks in her room in the middle of the night. In your examination you note that she is a quiet girl with a body weight below the 85th percentile but otherwise there are no obvious medical problems that could be attributed to her weight loss. Her history also reveals that her last menstrual period was six months ago. The most likely cause of her amenorrhea is:

A. Constitutional delay

B. Hyperthyroidism

C. Hypothyroidism

D. Hypothalamic dysfunction

E. Karyotype abnormality

107. A 34-year-old female smoker on oral contraceptive pills develops dyspnea, tachypnea, shortness of breath, chest pain, and hemoptysis two days after an intramedullary nailing of a severely comminuted left femur fracture. A spiral CT reveals a large embolus in the middle lobe of the right lung. The factor that probably contributed most to development of this embolus is:

A. Oral contraceptive use

B. Smoking

C. Femur fracture and surrounding tissue damage

D. DIC

E. SLE

108. A 74-year-old white male is diagnosed with prostate cancer with metastatic lesions present in the vertebral bodies. His physician is suggesting androgen deprivation therapy. Which of the following best characterizes the mechanism of action of antiandrogen flutamide?

A. Analog of GnRH

B. 5-alpha reductase inhibitor

C. Competitively inhibits androgens at testosterone receptor

D. Inhibition of steroid synthesis

E. Promotes rapid hydrolysis of testosterone

109. A 26-year-old woman presents to her physician because she has not had a menstrual period in more than six months. In addition, she reports a milky discharge from her breasts and decreased interest in sex for the last six months. A pregnancy test is negative. An excess of which of the following hormones is most likely responsible for her symptoms.

A. Adrenocorticotropin hormone (ACTH)

B. Prolactin (PRL)

C. Luteinizing hormone (LH)

D. Growth hormone (GH)

110. A major difference between *Haemophilus influenzae* and *Staphylococcus aureus* is:

A. *H. influenzae* causes pneumonia.

B. *S. aureus* can be life threatening.

C. *S. aureus* has a plasmid.

D. *H. influenzae* has a thin peptidoglycan layer and a phospholipid bilayer.

E. *S. aureus* has a capsule.

111. A 58-year-old woman with sialolithiasis is scheduled for a parotidectomy on the right side. The surgeon must take special care to avoid which of the following structures during the surgery?

A. Facial artery

B. Trigeminal nerve

C. Facial nerve

D. Auriculotemporal nerve

E. Lingual artery

112. A 6-year-old boy of Jewish descent comes to your clinic for the first time. His mother states that he was diagnosed with cystic fibrosis when he was 4 years old. Which of the following nutritional deficiencies would you be most suspect of?

A. Vitamin B_1

B. Vitamin B_{12}

C. Vitamin E

D. Folate

E. Niacin

113. A 68-year-old female has just found out that she has ovarian cancer and is expected to live only six more months. She expresses that this diagnosis must be wrong and that she will live. What stage is this patient in and what is the typical order of the stages this patient will likely go through in response to her imminent death?

    A. denial, bargaining, anger, depression, acceptance

    B. bargaining, denial, anger, depression, acceptance

    C. denial, depression, bargaining, anger, acceptance

    D. denial, anger, bargaining, depression, acceptance

    E. anger, denial, bargaining, acceptance, depression

114. A 21-year-old woman of Ashkenazi Jewish descent presents with diarrhea, crampy abdominal pain, and fever for the past four weeks. This is the second time she has suffered these symptoms. Her gastroenterologist suspects Crohn's disease. Which of the following best applies to Crohn's disease? **See Figure 114.**

    A. The anus is always affected.

    B. On gross pathology, pseudopolyps are frequently encountered.

    C. On gross pathology, noncaseating granulomas are frequently encountered.

    D. Toxic megacolon is a possible complication.

    E. There is a marked increase in the risk of developing colon cancer.

115. After unsuccessfully attempting to lower his total and LDL cholesterol levels through diet and exercise, a patient presents to your office for pharmacological management of his hyperlipidemia. You decide to start him on a drug from the class that affects the rate-limiting step in cholesterol synthesis. The drug that you would start and the lab tests you would periodically monitor throughout therapy are:

    A. Cholestyramine and liver function tests

    B. Niacin and renal function tests

    C. Niacin and liver function tests

    D. Lovastatin and liver function tests

    E. Gemfibrozil and prothrombin levels

116. A 55-year-old laboratory technician presents with a history of progressive dementia, dysarthria, muscle wasting, myoclonus, and athetosis. Autopsy diagnosis was Creutzfeldt-Jakob disease. This disease is caused by which of the following:

    A. Inborn error of metabolism

    B. Latent cytomegalovirus infection in an immunocompromised host

    C. Helminth infection

    D. Prion infection

    E. This disorder is idiopathic.

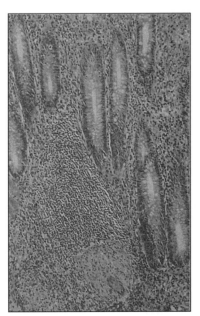

Figure 114 Reproduced with permission from Axford. Medicine. Blackwell Science, Ltd., 1996.

117. The friends of a 45-year-old man are concerned about his recent gradual changes in mental status and new onset "pill-rolling" tremor. His medical history includes chronic hepatitis. He is icteric, and slit-lamp examination of his eyes demonstrates green-gray Kayser-Fleischer rings. Clinical suspicion points to Wilson's disease and is corroborated by MRI exhibiting hepatolenticular degeneration and serum chemistries of elevated serum copper and decreased ceruloplasmin. Which of this following **(see Figure 117)** would most likely be his family pedigree?

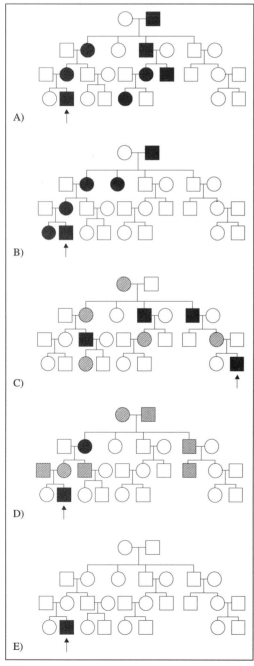

118. A 58-year-old obese man presents to his primary care physician "sick of being tired all the time." Recently remarried, his new wife is with him and states she cannot sleep in the same room as the patient because of his loud snoring. Which of the following is most accurate about the likely diagnosis?

A. More common in females

B. Treatment option is CPAP (continuous positive airway pressure)

C. Associated with cataplexy

D. Commonly associated with systemic or pulmonary hypotension

E. Stimulant drugs are the treatment of choice

119. An 18-year-old woman with body-mass index (BMI) of 20 presented with chest pains on exertion. Because the patient reported a family history of early-adulthood myocardial infarcts, the patient was thoroughly evaluated and later found to have severe coronary artery disease. The patient was immediately started on a low-fat diet, along with lovastatin. Which process is inhibited by lovastatin?

A. Inhibition of lipolysis in adipose tissue

B. Increase activity of lipoprotein lipase, thereby facilitating serum VLDL removal

C. Bind bile salts in the small intestine, preventing enterohepatic recirculation

D. Increase LDL uptake without upregulating LDL receptors

E. Inhibit the rate-limiting step in cholesterol synthesis

120. A 72-year-old woman complains of a fixed neck mass, dysphagia, hoarseness, and dyspnea. A biopsy was performed, and the result suggests a malignant tumor. She underwent surgery to remove the thyroid mass, and the recovery was unremarkable except for continuation of hoarseness. Which muscles are innervated by the recurrent laryngeal nerve?

   I. Aryepiglottic muscles
  II. Cricothyroid muscles
 III. Lateral cricoarytenoid muscles
  IV. Platysma muscles
   V. Thyroarytenoid muscles
  VI. Transverse arytenoid muscles

A. I, II, III, IV

B. II, III, IV, V

C. III, IV, V, VI

D. I, III, IV, V

E. I, III, V, VI

Figure 117

121. A 10-year-old boy in Columbus, Ohio, had a "cold" that lingered. He presented with shortness of breath, rales, and an enlarged liver. He is suspected of having myocarditis. He has no significant medical or travel history. Which of the following is the likely etiology?

    A. Coronavirus
    B. Coxsackie B virus
    C. *Trypanosoma cruzi*
    D. *Salmonella* sp.
    E. *Nocardia asteroides*

122. A resident attends a lecture about a patient he is going to be assigned. In the lecture, the cardiac surgeon states that in heart transplant patients, they usually do not reconnect the new heart to its nervous system connections. The surgeon then asks the resident to write a note to the nursing staff outlining what medications cannot be used on this patient in a cardiac emergency. Of the following medicines, which one would have the least beneficial effect in a heart transplant patient?

    A. Lidocaine
    B. Digitalis
    C. Amiodarone
    D. Adenosine
    E. Atropine

123. A 65-year-old man presented with bright red blood per rectum with his bowel movements. A full work-up included a colonoscopy, which was positive for an adenocarcinoma of the splenic colon. The tumor was treated with surgical removal of the involved section of colon. Postoperatively, serum levels of which of the following tumor markers should be followed to survey for possible recurrence of the patient's cancer?

    A. PSA
    B. CEA
    C. Alpha-fetoprotein
    D. CA-125
    E. S-100

124. A 55-year-old male patient is seen by his private medical doctor for abdominal pain. The patient has been vomiting for two days and unable to eat or drink. The patient's vital signs include a respiratory rate of 12 breaths per minute and a blood pressure of 116/78 mm Hg. The patient's pulse is tachycardic. When the patient goes from a supine to erect position, the blood pressure drops to

100/72 mm Hg with a rise in the pulse of 10 beats per minute. Lab results are as follows:

Na^+:	140 meq/L
K^+:	3.2 meq/L
Cl^-:	100 meq/L
PaO_2:	76 mm Hg
$PaCO_2$:	44 mm Hg

What is the best interpretation of this patient's acid-base disturbance?

    A. Metabolic acidosis
    B. Respiratory acidosis
    C. Metabolic alkalosis
    D. Respiratory alkalosis
    E. Mixed acid-base disorder

125. A 33-year-old woman with a recent history of heroin addiction is attending a drug treatment clinic. You are considering treatment of her addiction with another drug commonly used in heroin addicts. Which of the following pharmacologic principles best illustrates the practice of using this drug to treat heroin addiction?

    A. Therapeutic index
    B. Withdrawal
    C. Elimination
    D. Paradoxical reaction
    E. Cross-dependence

126. A 20-year-old woman with hypercholesterolemia was found to be unresponsive to lovastatin or other medications of the same class. Her total cholesterol levels were on the order of several thousand. The molecular basis for her condition was found to be two nonfunctional alleles of the LDL receptor. Over the next two years, she suffered multiple myocardial infarcts. Her prognosis for long-term survival was very poor.

She volunteered for a new gene therapy trial in which the cDNA for a functionally normal LDL receptor would be delivered to her hepatocytes. Which of the following gene delivery methods would provide efficient *permanent* lasting expression of the LDL gene?

    A. Retrovirus
    B. Liposomes
    C. Adenovirus
    D. Microinjection of DNA into the patient's liver cells
    E. Injection of an LDL-gene-bearing phage into the hepatic portal circulation

127. A 25-year-old gay male presents to your office with weight loss, a history of diarrhea, cough, and fever. On examination you see some reddish skin lesions. Which of the following drugs would you not treat him with?

A. Zidovudine

B. Amantadine

C. Saquinavir

D. Delavirdine

E. Didanosine

128. You are asked to see a 45-year-old male in the ER. He is a known alcoholic and a frequent visitor to the ER. This time, he is complaining of feeling hot and coughing up dark red, thick sputum. On physical examination, the patient has dullness to percussion at the lower right base. You decide to get a chest x-ray, which shows consolidation in the right lower lung field. A sputum Gram's stain shows many PMNs and gram-negative, encapsulated bacteria. What organism is likely to be responsible?

A. *Staphylococcus aureus*

B. *Klebsiella pneumoniae*

C. *Streptococcus pneumoniae*

D. *Mycoplasma*

E. *Pneumocystis carinii*

129. During a routine pelvic exam, you feel a mass that appears to be anterior to the vaginal wall. Which of the following structures are you likely to be feeling?

A. Perineal body

B. Bladder

C. Infundibulum

D. Ureter

E. Anterior fiber of the levator ani muscle

130. A 35-year-old woman was brought to the ER for sudden onset of nausea, vomiting, and severe abdominal cramps that radiate to the back. On physical exam, she is mildly obese with a temperature of 101°F and BP of 90/60. She has guarding of the abdomen with extreme tenderness to palpation in the epigastric area. Laboratory data shows elevated levels of serum amylase and lipase. Despite medical management, her conditions worsened over the next few days, and eventually she passed away. An autopsy was performed, and the pathologist found:

A. Caseous necrosis of the appendix

B. Gangrenous necrosis of the gallbladder

C. Fatty necrosis of the pancreas

D. Liquefactive necrosis of the lungs

E. None of the above

131. A middle-aged gentleman undergoes thyroid surgery to remove a nonmalignant thyroid nodule. During postoperative recovery, he begins to have abdominal cramps, paresthesia of the extremities, and muscle fasciculation. On physical exam, he has muscle twitching on tapping anterior to the tragus of the ear. What is the most likely abnormality?

A. Hypocalcemia

B. Hypokalemia

C. Hyponatremia

D. Hypomagnesemia

132. A 42-year-old female presents to the ER complaining of one week of mild bleeding from her gums that doesn't stop. She also complains of bruises on her thighs without trauma and minor vaginal bleeding even though she is not due to have her menstrual period for two more weeks. On exam, she has multiple ecchymoses on her legs and arms and petechiae on her calves. Her admission labs are (see Table 132):

Currently, the patient has minor gingival bleeding, but vital signs are stable. The patient denies taking any medications and has no significant past medical history. The best initial management for this patient is:

A. Prednisone

B. Intravenous immunoglobulin

C. Desmopressin

D. Vitamin K injection

E. Protamine sulfate

Table 132

CBC

WBC	9600/ul
Hb	12 g/dL
Hct	36.4%
Platelets	20,000/ul

SMA-7

Na	141 mEq/L
K	4.8 mEq/L
Cl	110 mEq/L
Bicarbonate	28 mEq/L
BUN	8.1 mg/dL
Creatinine	0.6 mg/dL
Glucose	96 mg/dL

Coags.

PT	16 s
INR	1.03
aPTT	34 s

133. A 41-year-old man is admitted to the hospital because of several days of jaundice. The patient states he had an episode of fevers, nausea, and anorexia about three weeks ago, but it resolved. Since then, he has had only mild fatigue, until developing jaundice recently. After a series of blood tests, his doctor tells him that he has an acute infection with hepatitis B. Which of the following sets of serum markers led the doctor to this diagnosis?

	HBsAg	HBeAg	IgM anti-coreAg	IgG anti-coreAg	anti-HBsAg
A.	–	–	–	–	+
B.	–	–	–	+	+
C.	+	+	–	+	–
D.	+	+	+	–	–
E.	+	–	–	+	–

134. A 2-year-old male is brought to the emergency room because of a chronic cough productive of thick green sputum. His parents report that he has been admitted to the hospital on six previous occasions for pneumonia. In addition, he has frequent, bulky, foul-smelling stools and was unable to defecate after birth due to a thick meconium plug. His weight is at the second percentile and height at the fifth percentile for his age. This child's disease is most likely related to which of the following genetic defects?

A. Deficiency of phenylalanine hydroxylase
B. Deficiency of lactase
C. Defective chloride ion channels
D. Defective potassium ion channels

135. Having more free time after your STEP 1 exam, you decide to get a new puppy. Knowing the various patterns of reinforcement, your goal is to train your puppy to sit, using treats as rewards. Which of the following reinforcement patterns would you choose based on its being the most difficult to extinguish?

A. Continuous reinforcement
B. Modeling
C. Variable reinforcement
D. Fixed reinforcement
E. All are equally difficult to extinguish

136. A 45-year-old obese white man comes to your office as a new patient. He needs a refill of one of his medications, which he ran out of several days ago; "A blood pressure medication" he notes, but doesn't recall the specific name. His vitals are as follows: HR 64, BP 155/95, RR 13, Temp. 37.2°C. His history reveals that he has type II diabetes mellitus, grade two cardiac heart failure, and general anxiety disorder. His BUN/Cr ratio is 14/1.2. Which of the following medications would you prescribe?

A. Beta-blocker
B. ACE inhibitor
C. Alpha-blocker
D. Diuretic
E. Calcium channel blocker

137. A 35-year-old male patient presents with shortness of breath, coughing, and some hemoptysis. History reveals that the patient is a well-known spelunker who has traveled all over the world. He grew up in the Mississippi River area. His chest x-ray that shows a cavitation in the right upper lobe. What is the most likely cause of his disease?

A. Primary tuberculosis

B. Secondary tuberculosis

C. *Blastomyces dermatitidis*

D. *Aspergillus fumigatus*

E. *Histoplasma capsulatum*

138. A 32-year-old African American man is started on trimethoprim/sulfamethoxazole (Bactrim) for an upper respiratory infection. A few days later, he develops fatigue and jaundice. Laboratory tests indicate the presence of a mild hemolytic anemia. Further testing is likely to show an inherited deficiency in which of the following enzymes?

A. Glucose-6-phosphate dehydrogenase

B. Pyruvate kinase

C. Phosphofructokinase

D. Phosphoglycerate kinase

139. Which of the following ranks psychosocial stressors from most to least severe?

A. Divorce, being fired, beginning or ending formal schooling

B. Death of child, change in residence, serious medical illness

C. Birth of first child, spouse's death, marriage

D. Death of close friend, change in residence, marital separation

E. Marital separation, trouble with boss, detention in jail

140. A 35-year-old white female presents to your office for the first time. She has been reading about thyroid cancer in a popular women's magazine and is very concerned that she may have thyroid cancer. She has no history of exposure to ionizing radiation or of residing in an area of iodine deficiency. Physical examination is entirely within normal limits. When you try to assure her, she persists in asking about different thyroid cancers. Which of the following would be correct to tell her?

A. Follicular carcinoma is most common, present at a younger age compared to papillary carcinoma, increased in areas of iodine deficiency; usually a cold nodule

B. Papillary carcinomas are associated with previous exposure to ionizing radiation. Psammoma bodies may be present within selected lesions

C. Medullary carcinomas are derived from C cells, In some cases they may also release VIP; medullary carcinoma is associated with MEN-I

D. Anaplastic carcinoma occurs mainly in young patients; they may have a microscopic appearance similar to small cell carcinoma

141. In the cardiac cycle, which of the follow statements are true:

I. During isovolumetric contraction, blood is not ejected by the ventricles.

II. During isovolumetric relaxation, ventricular filling occurs.

III. Blood volume in the ventricles at the beginning of isovolumetric relaxation is equal to the end diastolic volume.

IV. Stroke volume is EDV (end diastolic volume) − ESV (end systolic volume).

A. I, II

B. I, IV

C. I, II, IV

D. II, III, IV

E. I, II, III, IV

142. A 19-year-old female is rushed to the ER by her brother. Her boyfriend just broke up with her. In a suicide attempt she took an unknown amount of Tylenol (acetaminophen) and aspirin. You order the appropriate labs, psychiatry consult, and close monitoring of her vital signs. Which antidote would you administer?

A. Acetylcysteine

B. Dimercaprol

C. Naloxone

D. Penicillamine

E. Deferoxamine

143. A mother brings her 12-year-old son to you because of loose, greasy diarrhea that seemed to have started after a Scout hike during which he may have drunk from a stream. The stools have a very foul-smelling odor but no blood. You take a specimen finding trophozoites and some cysts. The cause of this child's diarrhea is:

A. *Giardia lamblia*

B. *Entamoeba histolytica*

C. *Cryptosporidium*

D. *Trichomonas vaginalis*

E. *Balantidium*

144. A 4-month-old boy is seen on rounds with a history of fever and hypertension. On ophthalmic exam, he is noted to have corneal opacities like his sister. Other than small, dark red lesions on his genitals, abdomen, and buttocks, his abdominal exam is unremarkable. Which of the following enzymes is most likely deficient?

A. α-Galactosidase

B. α-Hexosaminidase A

C. α-Glucosidase

D. β-Galactosidase

E. α-Hexosaminidase A and B

145. A 26-year-old woman presents to her primary care physician complaining of nightmares and flashbacks of a severe car accident that took place six months ago. She now is afraid to drive and has intense anxiety when she gets in her car. She also reports poor concentration and being very irritable. Which of the following is the most likely diagnosis?

A. Specific phobia

B. Malingering

C. Dissociative disorder

D. Posttraumatic stress disorder (PTSD)

E. Normal reaction

146. A 20-year-old male, short-stature patient on the psychiatric unit requires a pulmonary consultation for new onset of productive cough. The patient has a history of repeated chest infections. The patient indicates having multiple upper respiratory chest infections and has been hospitalized once this year for productive cough with purulent sputum. You diagnose a mild genetic form of cystic fibrosis with electrolyte sweat testing. Sputum cultures confirm the presence of a gram-negative bacillus. Which cephalosporin would be the best choice for coverage against these gram-negative bacilli?

A. Cefoxitin

B. Cefepime

C. Cefixime

D. Ceftriaxone

E. Cefaclor

147. A 55-year-old Caucasian male with lung cancer has been informed that his malignancy has metastasized to the brain and that his median survival time is nine months. On a followup, the patient returns to the physician's office with his wife. When given treatment options, the patient states "I don't know what to do, ask my wife." The wife confides in the physician that since his diagnosis, her husband has become almost childlike, depending on her to make all decisions. What defense mechanism is the patient displaying?

A. Sublimation

B. Denial

C. Suppression

D. Repression

E. Regression

148. A Hispanic male migrant farm worker is brought to the clinic by his wife of 25 years. His wife states that he has had a productive cough for more than three weeks, with chest pain and hemoptysis. She states he awakens at night with fever and chills that "soak his shirt." He has started to lose weight and finds it difficult to continue working because of fatigue. The patient does not smoke, does not use alcohol, and denies any illegal drug use. In viewing the chest x-ray, abnormalities are seen in the upper lobe segments of the lung. **See Figure 148.** Restriction fragment length polymorphism (RFLP) testing isolates the specific strain of the patient's infection, and you begin treatment. One of the key agents in the treatment commonly produces peripheral neuropathy, dermatitis, and diarrhea. These side effects can be reversed with the administration of which vitamin?

A. Vitamin A
B. Vitamin B_{12}
C. Vitamin C
D. Vitamin B_6
E. Vitamin E

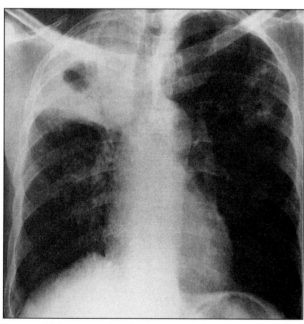

Figure 148   Reproduced with permission from Armstrong. Diagnostic Imaging, 4/e. Blackwell Science, Ltd., 1998.

149. You are on the ambulance that responds to an anxious 29-year-old woman in the ninth month of her second pregnancy. She suddenly begins to have vaginal bleeding. She states that the painless, bright red bleeding started 1.5 hours ago. Your physical examination reveals an anxious patient with cool, clammy skin who is pale with peripheral cyanosis. The patient's pulse is 130, blood pressure is 80/60, and respirations are 28. The fetal heart sounds can be auscultated. What is the most accurate definition of her status?

A. A state where metabolic needs increase with a rapid decrease in arterial blood pH
B. A state where the level of carbon dioxide in the blood exceeds 60 mm Hg
C. A state where cells become less permeable, which prevents oxygen from being transported into the cells
D. A state of inadequate tissue perfusion with oxygen and nutrients
E. A state of decreased urinary output and increased serum glucose levels

150. A 54-year-old male presents to the ER while you are on duty. He complains of right knee pain so intense that "Even a sheet cannot touch my leg!" After history and physical exam you decide to aspirate the joint. You send the yellow cloudy fluid for culture, stain, review for crystals and make a slide for yourself. The slide you view has needle-shaped crystals that are negatively birefringent. Which of the following drugs would you select to treat this patient?

A. Xanthine oxidase inhibitors
B. Indomethacin
C. Uricosuric agents
D. Aspirin

BLOCK III - ANSWER KEY

101-B	114-C	127-B	139-A
102-C	115-D	128-B	140-B
103-E	116-D	129-B	141-B
104-C	117-D	130-C	142-A
105-D	118-B	131-A	143-A
106-D	119-E	132-A	144-A
107-C	120-E	133-D	145-D
108-C	121-B	134-C	146-B
109-B	122-E	135-C	147-E
110-D	123-B	136-B	148-D
111-C	124-C	137-E	149-D
112-C	125-E	138-A	150-B
113-D	126-A		

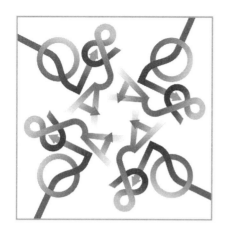

ANSWERS
BLOCK 3

101. B Kuru is caused by virulent proteins that cause improper folding of cytoplasmic prion proteins resulting in a vast accumulation of these proteins. This will lead to subacute spongiform encephalopathy which is characteristic of Kuru.

A. Progressive multifocal leukoencephalopathy is caused by the JC virus. It is a disease that causes problems in immunosuppressed people and principally affects the white matter. It has no effect on protein folding.

C. Rabies is caused by the rabies virus. It is spread by the bites of rabid animals and causes degeneration of neurons in the brain stem. This has no effect on protein folding.

D. Measles virus also causes viral encephalitis and leads to a special condition called subacute sclerosing panencephalitis. It is a virus and has no effect on protein folding.

E. Dengue results in bone pain, rash, fever, muscle pain, and headache. It is caused by the dengue virus, which has no effect protein folding.

102. C Prednisone is a glucocorticoid associated with hypocalcemia because it decreases calcium absorption from the intestines and from the renal tubules. It does increase PTH mediated bone reabsorption; however, there is still a net negative Ca++ balance.

A. Prednisone has mineralocorticoid activity and will stimulate water retention and weight gain.

B. Prednisone has aldosteronelike activity where Na is reabsorbed and K+/H+ is secreted, resulting in hypokalemia. While it is possible that ibuprofen might result in hyperkalemia through a mechanism

of reducing renal blood flow and worsening renal function, it is not likely.

D. NSAIDs and glucocorticoids do not cause liver toxicity.

E. Glucocorticoids lead to polycythemia, not anemia.

103. E Scaphoid fractures are at high risk of developing AVN because the blood supply is so tenuous. The distal one-third of the bone has no direct blood supply so if separated from the proximal two-thirds it can easily necrose. The risk of AVN with scaphoid fractures is quite significant and these fractures must always be diagnosed to prevent this dreaded complication.

A, B, C, and **D** are all incorrect because the blood supply to these bones is adequate and fractures of these bones rarely result in AVN.

104. C The disease in this case is acute intermittent porphyria (AIP). AIP occurs as a result of a deficiency in uroporphyrinogen synthase, an enzyme found in the heme synthesis pathway. Certain conditions such as hypoxia and certain drugs such as rifampin and barbiturates can induce the synthesis of cytochrome P-450 in the liver, a molecule that utilizes heme in its structure. This depletes the supply of heme, which disinhibits ALA synthase (the first enzyme in the heme synthesis pathway) thereby causing a buildup of the metabolites that precede the deficient enzyme, ultimately resulting in an acute attack. The metabolites responsible for the symptoms are delta-aminolevulinate (ALA) and porphobilinogen (PBG), which can be measured in the urine. These metabolites, acting upon the nervous system, cause the symptoms seen in this disease. Visceral pain fibers are excited and cause the abdominal pain. Autonomic nerves are disrupted and can result in constipation, tachycardia, and/or increased blood pressure. Peripheral nerve disruption may cause muscle weakness, sensory loss, and/or parasthesias. Cerebral involvement can imitate psychiatric conditions, resulting in symptoms of depression, anxiety, agitation, paranoia, and confusion. Seizures are even possible. If these symptoms are misinterpreted as reflecting a psychiatric or primary seizure disorder, treatment with sedative-hypnotics, tranquilizers, and/or anticonvulsants will worsen the symptoms and jeopardize the patient's life.

A. This enzyme, found in the metabolism of the sulfur-containing amino acids methionine and cysteine, converts homocysteine to cystathionine. A deficiency causes homocystinuria, resulting in osteoporosis, increased length and decreased thickness of the long bones, lens dislocation, cardiovascular complications in childhood (deep vein thrombosis, atherosclerosis, stroke), and mental retardation.

B. This enzyme is involved simultaneously in both the metabolism of folate and homocysteine. This enzyme "untraps" the storage form of folate (methyl-tetrahydrofolate) by converting it to tetrahydrofolate, this form being able to enter into the synthesis of purines as well as the pyrimidine thymidine. The enzyme does this by removing the methyl group from the storage form of THF and putting it onto homocysteine, thereby creating free THF and methionine. A deficiency in this enzyme therefore would result in a buildup of homocysteine, causing homocystinuria, described above in the explanation for answer A.

D. This enzyme converts homogentisic acid to maleylacetoacetate, a deficiency of which results in a build up of homogentisic acid and resultant alcaptonuria. This disease causes dark urine, ochronosis (darkly pigmented cartilage), and arthritis in older patients (due to buildup of this metabolite in the joints).

E. and F. These enzymes are involved in the breakdown of branched-chain ketoacids (which were derived from the branched-chain amino acids valine, leucine, and isoleucine). These amino acids are transaminated in skeletal muscle and transported to the liver as alpha-ketoacids. In the liver the first enzyme, branched-chain ketoacid dehydrogenase, oxidatively decarboxylates all three ketoacids. A deficiency in this enzyme causes maple syrup urine disease. A complete deficiency causes severe mental retardation, acidosis, lethargy, periods of hypertonia alternating with hypotonia, sweet-smelling urine, coma, and, if treatment is unsuccessful, early death. The enzyme mentioned in answer choice F, methylmalonyl-CoA mutase, is the last enzyme of a pathway common to valine and isoleucine, but not leucine. The leucine pathway diverts from the valine and isoleucine pathways just after the branched-chain ketoacid dehydrogenase step, leucine eventually being converted into acetyl-Coa. Methylmalonyl-CoA mutase converts methymalonyl-CoA into succinyl-CoA. A deficiency of this enzyme causes a buildup of methylmalonic acid in the blood and urine (methylmalonic aciduria), causing a life-threatening acidosis, as well as neurotoxicity, in the infant.

105. D The clinical picture of rising pCO_2, decreased wheezing (likely indicating decreased air movement due to increasing bronchoconstriction), and continued respiratory distress indicates fatigue of respiratory muscles that may require intubation.

A. The increase in CO_2 indicates that the patient is now unable to "blow off" CO_2 at the rate she previously could, an ominous sign.

B. Decreased wheezing on physical examination can be paradoxical in asthma, as it may correspond to decreased air movement due to further (near total) bronchoconstriction.

C. Although steroids exert some immediate effects, their main actions (alterations in protein synthesis) require several hours to produce improvement in symptoms.

106. D This patient is suffering from anorexia nervosa, characterized by a refusal to maintain body weight over the 85th percentile, restriction of food intake, and amenorrhea. Hypothalamic dysfunction can result from low body fat and a body weight below the 85th percentile that results in either primary or, as in this case, secondary amenorrhea.

A. Constitutional delay is a form of primary amenorrhea. This patient has had periods in the past, but they have ceased due to weight loss and hypothalamic dysfunction.

B. Hyperthyroidism is a cause of menstrual abnormalities including amenorrhea, however patients with hyperthyroidism complain of decreased weight in the presence of an increased appetite and food intake. The patient was not found to have any of the signs or symptoms of hyperthyroidism: exophthalmos, anxiety, tremors, tachycardia, or goiter.

C. Hypothyroidism is a cause of menstrual abnormalities that includes amenorrhea and also polymenorrhea (cycles lasting less than 21 days). Other signs and symptoms of hypothyroidism include weight gain, weakness and lethargy, cold intolerance, dry/brittle hair and skin, and depression.

E. Karyotype abnormalities, such as Turner's syndrome (XO), cause primary amenorrhea due to gonadal dysgenesis.

107. C Severe tissue damage is considered a major risk factor for the development of a thromboembolus. The soft tissue damage sustained in a comminuted femur fracture as well as the actual bone injury itself is usually quite severe and the most likely factor of those listed above to cause a pulmonary embolus. Any major trauma that results in significant tissue injury greatly increases the risk of clot formation.

A. Oral contraceptive use does increase the risk of thrombosis but not nearly as much as in the case described above.
B. Smoking does increase the risk of pulmonary embolus but not nearly as much as the femur fracture and nailing.
D. Although DIC can very easily lead to pulmonary embolus development, the description given in the question does not fit DIC.
E. There is no reason to suspect systemic lupus erythematosus, though SLE usually leads to a hypercoagulable state.

108. C Flutamide is an antiandrogen used in the treatment of prostate carcinomas. It works at the testosterone receptor and mechanism of action is competitive inhibition of androgens.

A. Leuprolide is the antiandrogen, which is a GnRH analog.
B. Finasteride is the antiandrogen with a mechanism of 5-alpha reductase inhibition.
D. Antiandrogens such as ketoconazole inhibit steroid synthesis.
E. This is not a mechanism of action of an antiandrogen.

109. B This patient has the classic symptoms of hyperprolactinemia, the most common pituitary hormone hypersecretion syndrome. PAL-secreting pituitary adenomas cause oligo- or amenorrhea, galactorrhea, vaginal dryness, and loss of libido. After ruling out pregnancy and other physiologic causes for elevated prolactin levels, a pituitary MRI can confirm the presence of an adenoma. Bromocriptine, a dopamine agonist, can be used to treat prolactinomas.

A. Elevated ACTH levels cause Cushing's syndrome, characterized by central obesity, moon facies, thin skin, purple striae, and other stigmata.
C. LH-secreting tumors are very rare, presenting more often with optic chiasm pressure.

D. GH-secreting adenomas cause acromegaly, characterized by frontal bossing, increased hand and foot size, and mandibular enlargement.

110. D *H. influenzae* is a gram-negative bacteria that has two phospholipid bilayers with a thin peptidoglycan layer separating them. *S. aureus* is a gram-positive bacteria with a thick peptidoglycan layer and a phospholipid bilayer underneath.

A. *S. aureus* can also cause a bacteremia that is also manifested by pneumonia.
B. *S. aureus* causes toxic shock syndrome and *H. influenzae* causes meningitis and pneumonia, all of which are life threatening.
C. All bacteria store DNA in plasmids.
E. Both *S. aureus* and *H. influenzae* have capsules.

111. C The facial nerve runs under and around the parotid gland and is always at high risk of injury during parotid surgery. **See Figure 111.**

A. The facial artery is found well inferior to the parotid at the angle of the mandible.
B. The trigeminal nerve branches deep within the skull a great distance from the parotid.
D. This nerve is found well posterior to the parotid.
E. The lingual artery is found inferior and deep to the parotid.

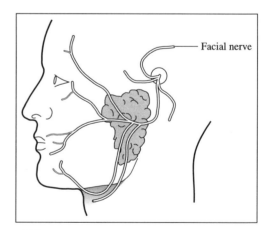

Figure 111

112. C Patients with cystic fibrosis have a plethora of problems, most of which involve the respiratory tract as they have difficulty expectorating thick mucoid secretions due to the abnormal CFTR gene. In addition, they have problems with their pancreas since it functions as an endocrine and exocrine gland and can also be obstructed by secretions. Because the pancreas secretes lipase, an enzyme necessary for the digestion and absorption of fats, this function may be compromised in patients with cystic fibrosis. As a result, a patient with cystic fibrosis can be susceptible to malabsorption of fat-soluble vitamins. Therefore, the correct answer is C, vitamin E, since it is the only fat-soluble vitamin of the choices. All the remaining choices are water-soluble vitamins and can easily cross the lumen. Although B_{12} requires intrinsic factor for absorption, this is not a problem in patients with cystic fibrosis.

113. D The initial reaction to dying is often denial, in which the patient refuses to believe a diagnosis. This is often followed by anger when the patient realizes his/her impending death. The next stage is often a bargaining period, in which the patient attempts to bargain for more time. Next, the patient experiences depression when the realization of death occurs. Finally, the patient will typically experience acceptance of his/her death.

A, B, C, and **E** are all incorrect.

114. C Crohn's disease is characterized grossly by "creeping fat," noncaseating granulomas, cobblestone appearance of the intestinal lumen, and fissures with fistulae formation. Any part of the GI tract, from the mouth to the anus, may be affected. **See Table 114.**

A. The anus is not often affected in Crohn's disease.

B. Pseudopolyps are found in ulcerative colitis.

D. Toxic megacolon is a complication of UC, rarely found in Crohn's disease.

E. In Crohn's, the risk of colon cancer is small. However, in ulcerative colitis, the risk of colon cancer is significantly increased.

115. D Statins are the class of drugs that lower plasma cholesterol by inhibiting HMG-CoA reductase, the rate-limiting step in cholesterol synthesis. They undergo first-pass extraction by the liver, and can cause biochemical abnormalities in liver function. Therefore, periodic monitoring of liver function testing is advised.

A. Cholestyramine is a bile acid binding resin. No lab tests are necessary.

B. Niacin inhibits lipolysis in adipose tissue and decreases liver triacylglycerol synthesis. Hepatotoxicity has been reported, so liver function tests, not renal function tests, should be performed.

C. Niacin inhibits lipolysis in adipose tissue and decreases liver triacylglycerol synthesis. Hepatotoxicity has been reported, so liver function tests should be performed.

E. Gemfibrizol is a fibrate that stimulates lipoprotein lipase activity. It is used to decrease plasma triacylglycerol levels. It competes with Coumadin for binding sites, so prothrombin levels should be monitored in patients taking both of these medications.

Table 114

	ULCERATIVE COLITIS	CROHN'S DISEASE
Infectious etiology?	No	Likely
Location	Isolated to colon	Anywhere in GI tract
Lesions	Contiguously proximal from colon	Skip lesions, disseminated
Inflammation	Limited to mucosa/submucosa	Transmural
Neoplasms	Very high risk for development	Lower risk for development
Fissures	None	Extend through submucosa
Fistula	None	Frequent: can be enterocutaneous
Granulomas	None	Noncaseating are characteristic
Extraintestinal manifestations	Seen in both: • Arthritis, iritis, erythema nodosum, pyoderma gangrenosum • Sclerosing cholangitis = chronic, fibrosing, inflammation of biliary system leading to cholestasis & portal hypertension	

Reproduced with permission from Ayala. Pathophysiology for the Boards and Wards. Blackwell Science, Inc., 2000.

116. D Proteinaceous infectious particles (prions) are the so-called "slow viruses," and are responsible for Creutzfeldt-Jakob disease, Kuru, scrapie (in sheep), and bovine spongiform encephalopathy ("mad cow disease"). Prions contain no genetic material (RNA or DNA), differentiating them from viruses. The agents are transmissible to humans or primates through brain or eye tissue. There is no cure for these infections, which follow a rapidly downhill course once they become clinically evident. The disease has been noted years after exposure to needles, instruments, or electrodes used in treatment or examination of an infected patient.

A. Creutzfeldt-Jakob disease is not an inborn error of metabolism, although vertical transmission of the infection does occur.

B. Creutzfeldt-Jakob disease is not a latent cytomegalovirus infection in an immunocompromised host.

C. Creutzfeldt-Jakob disease is not a helminthic infection.

E. Creutzfeldt-Jakob disease is caused by a prion.

117. D Wilson's disease is autosomal recessive.

A. This pedigree is autosomal dominant.

B. This pedigree is X-linked dominant.

C. This pedigree is X-linked recessive.

E. This pedigree is a spontaneous mutation.

118. B Sleep apnea is associated with obesity, loud snoring, arrhythmias, and even sudden death. More common in males, sleep apnea patients commonly present as being fatigued or tired during the day and may not know they are waking up during the night with apneic spells (diagnosis requires at least 10 seconds during sleep in which the individual stops breathing). It is classified as either central (no respiratory effort) or obstructive (continued respiratory effort usually against airway obstruction from excessive tissue).

A. Sleep apnea is more common in males than females.

C. Cataplexy (sudden loss of muscle tone) is associated with narcolepsy.

D. Sleep apnea is seen often with concomitant systemic or pulmonary hypertension.

E. Treatments include weight loss, CPAP, antidepressant therapy if indicated (depression is often a comorbidity), and surgery if indicated. Stimulants are indicated for narcolepsy.

119. E Lovastatin is a 3-hydroxy-3-methylglutarate-CoA (HMG–CoA) reductase inhibitor, an inhibitor of the rate-limiting step in cholesterol synthesis. These inhibitors ("statins") also, through a feedback mechanism, stimulate an increase in LDL-receptor expression.

A. Niacin is an inhibitor of adipose lipolysis.

B. Clofibrate increases lipoprotein lipase activity.

C. Bile salt-binding resins such as cholestyramine and colestipol interfere with enterohepatic recirculation.

D. Probucol upregulates a normally low-affinity LDL uptake mechanism without increasing LDL-receptor expression.

120. E Hürthle cell carcinomas are usually found in patients over the age of 60. Depending on the size and the location of the tumor, they have the potential to impinge on the recurrent laryngeal nerve, causing hoarseness and dysphagia. Biopsy is indicated for diagnosis. Treatment requires surgical resection because Hürthle cell carcinomas are radioresistant. The function of the recurrent laryngeal nerve depends on the malignancy of the tumor as well as the surgical risks of resection.

A. The cricothyroid muscles are innervated by the external laryngeal branch of the superior laryngeal branch of the vagus nerve, and they tense the vocal cords. The platysma muscles are innervated by the facial nerve, and they depress the lower jaw and lip and the angle of the mouth.

B. Both the thyroarytenoid muscles and the lateral cricoarytenoid muscles are innervated by the recurrent laryngeal nerve. They adduct and relax the vocal cords.

C. The transverse arytenoid muscles are innervated by the recurrent laryngeal nerve. They adduct and close the laryngeal inlet.

D. Aryepiglottic muscles are innervated by the recurrent laryngeal nerve. They adduct the vocal cords.

121. B Coxsackie B virus is a picornavirus that can cause myocardial and pericardial infections in both children and adults.

A. Coronavirus is the second most prevalent cause of the common cold. Its name is derived from the solar appearance of the virion caused by corona-like projections emanating from its surface, not any relation to the cardiovascular system.

C. *T. cruzi* is the causative organism of Chagas disease, which often involves the myocardium. However, this boy does not have a history of travel to Central or South America where this organism would be a likely etiology.

D. *Salmonella* sp. cause enteritis, septicemia, enteric fever, or an asymptomatic colonization but do not cause myocarditis.

E. *Nocardia* is a gram-positive organism that exhibits acid-fast staining. *N. asteroides* causes primarily bronchopulmonary or cutaneous infection in patients with chronic pulmonary disease, immunocompromise, or in whom the organism was introduced into subcutaneous tissue through trauma.

122. E Atropine would have no effect on a transplanted heart. For atropine to be effective, the vagus has to be connected to the heart. Without vagal innervation, atropine would have little cardiac effect.

A, B, C, and **D** are incorrect. They can all be used in cardiac transplant patients because their mechanism of action does not depend on the vagus.

123. B Carcinoembryonic antigen, CEA, serum level is used as a monitor of recurrence in colorectal neoplasms. Note that it is not appropriate as a screening tool, as other GI tumors may also elevate serum levels of this marker.

A. Prostate specific antigen, PSA, is used for evaluation of prostate cancer. Its use for prostate cancer screening is still somewhat controversial, though it is generally acceptable to use change in levels of PSA to follow prostate cancer progression.

C. Alpha-fetoprotein is used for evaluation of hepatocellular carcinoma as well as yolk sac tumors. CA-125 is used to monitor disease progression in ovarian cancer.

E. S-100 is used to evaluate malignant melanomas.

124. C Metabolic alkalosis occurs when there is an increased load of base in the body, such as when an elderly patient consumes too many antacids (milk-alkali syndrome) or when you lose too many hydrogen ions during prolonged vomiting. Intractable vomiting also worsens metabolic alkalosis. In addition to the loss of hydrogen ions, there is an associated volume depletion, as seen in this patient with positive orthostatic pressure changes. This triggers the renin-angiotensin-aldosterone system. Increased

aldosterone stimulates the reabsorption of H_2O via the Na^+/H^+ pump, which further reabsorbs bicarbonate ion in order to function properly, and the Na^+/K^+ pump, which causes a potassium depleted state. The values in this patient reflect these facts. Furthermore, the respiratory system compensates for the patient's simple metabolic alkalosis by creating an acidotic state via hypoventilation, allowing for CO_2 retention. This increases the $PaCO_2$ levels. It also decreases the PaO_2 since less ventilation equals less oxygenation.

A guide to follow in acid-base problems is to come up with an acid-base laboratory interpretation algorithm such as:

Evaluate	1. Consider patient history and the conditions that should be present
Remember	2. pH = HCO_3^- $PaCO_2$
Remember	3. Compensation always moves in the same direction as the primary disorder
Remember	4. pH always represents the primary disorder
Remember	5. A clue to the existence of a mixed acid-base disorder is a pH that is normal in the presence of abnormal H^+ & HCO_3^-
Evaluate	6. Arterial labs for $PaCO_2$ & HCO_3^- levels
Evaluate	7. pH levels
Evaluate	8. If disorder is partially compensated or uncompensated
Determine	9. Determine condition

A. Metabolic acidosis is a condition in which the body fluids become acidotic because of an increased load of organic acids in the body such as occurs in shock, diabetes, or renal failure.

B. Respiratory acidosis is a condition in which the body fluids become acidotic because of a failure in the respiratory system.

D. Respiratory alkalosis is a situation where CO_2 is blown off too rapidly by the lungs with a subsequent rise in serum pH.

E. Mixed acid-base disorder is revealed when bicarbonate and/or H^+ levels are abnormal but in the presence of a normal looking pH value.

125. E Methadone, a synthetic opiate, is used to treat heroin addiction and decrease the euphoria experienced when heroin is used. It can be substituted for heroin safely due to cross-dependence. Essentially an addiction to a less harmful substance (methadone) is substituted for addiction to illicit drugs. Methadone has a long half-life with a steadier bioavailability in contrast to the peaks and crashes of heroin use. It is an opiate receptor agonist and its action at these receptors blocks potential withdrawal symptoms when heroin use is stopped.

A. Therapeutic index refers to the ratio of toxic dose: effective dose.
B. Withdrawal phenomena occur upon discontinuation of a drug; methadone is administered to help prevent opioid withdrawal.
C. Elimination refers to removal of a drug from the body.
D. Paradoxical reactions occur when an administered medication results in an action opposite that which was intended (an example is when diphenhydramine (Benadryl) is prescribed for sleep but instead causes a patient to become more agitated and unable to sleep.

126. A A retrovirus is the only one of these methods that would provide permanent gene delivery to a large enough number of hepatocytes to help this patient. The retrovirus DNA, plus the gene of interest, would be integrated into the genome of the target cells, giving permanent expression.

B. Lipid vesicles only yield transient expression because the DNA remains episomal and not integrated into the chromosomes.
C. Like lipid vesicles, the gene therapy would only last transiently.
D. Microinjection is very inefficient as a means of transfer since it is performed at a cell-by-cell basis. Microinjection is best suited for germ-line (as opposed to somatic) gene therapy, should it ever be permitted.
E. Bacteriophages do not deliver DNA into mammalian cells, only into host bacteria.

127. B This patient has contracted HIV disease. Amantadine is used to treat influenza infection, not HIV infection.

A. Zidovudine (AZT) is a nucleoside reverse transcriptase inhibitor used in the treatment of HIV infection.
C. Saquinavir is a protease inhibitor used in the treatment of HIV infection.
D. Delaviridine is a nonnucleoside reverse transcriptase inhibitor used in the treatment of HIV infection.
E. Didanosine (ddI) is a nucleoside reverse transcriptase inhibitor used in the treatment of HIV infection.

128. B This patient has a fever, productive cough, and consolidation on chest x-ray, which are highly suggestive of pneumonia. The thick, red sputum is classically seen in *Klebsiella* pneumonia. *Klebsiella* is a frequent cause of pneumonia in alcoholics, as in this case, and diabetics. It is an encapsulated gram-negative rod.

A. *Staph aureus* is a gram-positive organism. It often causes pneumonia following a previous influenza episode.
C. *Strep pneumoniae* is the most common cause of community-acquired pneumonia. However, it is a gram-positive organism.
D. *Mycoplasmae* causes an atypical pneumonia, sometimes called a "walking pneumonia." Chest x-ray usually shows an interstitial infiltrate rather than a consolidation, and there would be no organisms seen on Gram's stain of the sputum.
E. *Pneumocystis* causes a pneumonia most often seen in AIDS patients. Again, the Gram's stain is inconsistent with *P. carinii* in this case.

129. B The bladder can be easily palpated anteriorly through the vaginal wall.

A. The perineal body is a posterior structure that separates the vagina from the rectum.
C. The infundibulum is the lateral end of the uterine tubes. The possibility of palpating these structures at all is remote.
D. The ureters are posterior-lateral to the vagina.
E. The levator ani muscles are lateral structures.

130. C Acute pancreatitis is an inflammatory episode with symptoms related to intrapancreatic activation of enzymes, i.e., amylase, lipase. Symptoms vary widely in severity, complications, and prognosis. Causes include gallstones, alcohol, trauma/surgery, medications (e.g., didanosine), metabolic (e.g., hypertriglyceridemia and hypercalcemia), infections, and scorpion venom. Pathological findings include autodigestion of the pancreas, interstitial edema, hemorrhage, and cell and fat necrosis. While most patients recover, the mortality is 3 to 5%.

A. Appendicitis classically presents with pain localized to RLQ (McBurney's point). Furthermore, caseous necrosis of the appendix is unlikely since the appendix does not have digestive enzymes.

B. Pain from cholecystitis can refer to the shoulder (Murphy's sign).

D. Lung involvement in this patient is unlikely, except in complications such as ARDS.

E. Incorrect.

131. A The patient exhibits signs of hypocalcemia which includes neuromuscular irritability, weakness, weight loss, diarrhea, bone pain, headache, seizures, and dry skin. Other signs include Chvostek's sign (exhibited in this patient) and Trousseau's sign (carpal spasm after inflation of a blood pressure cuff above the systolic pressure). Calcium level is controlled by parathyroid hormone (PTH) and calcitonin. PTH maintains calcium level by increasing bone resorption of calcium, increasing kidney reabsorption of calcium in the distal convoluted tubes, decreasing kidney reabsorption of phosphate, and increasing 1,25 $(OH)_2$ cholecalciferol production by stimulating kidney 1 α-hydroxylase. A decrease in free serum Ca^{2+} increases PTH secretion. An increase in serum Ca^{2+} increases calcitonin secretion. Calcitonin decreases bone resorption of calcium. Other causes of hypocalcemia include Addison's disease, carcinoma of the thyroid, malabsorption, and renal disease.

B. Potassium is a major electrolyte, and nearly 98% of the body's potassium is located intracellularly. Hypokalemia may occur in renal or GI losses, inadequate diet, transcellular shift (movement of potassium from serum into cells), and medications. Signs include palpitations, skeletal muscle weakness or cramping, paralysis, paresthesias, constipation, nausea or vomiting, abdominal cramping, polyuria, nocturia, psychosis, delirium, and depression.

C. Sodium is a major ion of the extracellular fluid. Serum sodium concentration and serum osmolarity normally are maintained under precise control by homeostatic mechanisms involving thirst, antidiuretic hormone (ADH), and renal handling of filtered sodium. Hyponatremia occurs when there is an inappropriate loss of fluid.

D. Magnesium is a major cation in the body and is the second most common intracellular cation after potassium. Causes of hypomagnesemia include dietary deficiency, decreased absorption, increased excretion, alcoholism, uremia, diuretics, parathyroid disease, and eclampsia. Clinical effects of hypomagnesemia are greatest in the CNS, neuromuscular, GI, and cardiac systems.

132. A This patient has the classic presentation of idiopathic thrombocytopenic purpura (ITP). This is an autoimmune disease of unknown etiology that is caused by destruction of platelets by platelet antibodies. It is characterized by bleeding from mucosal surfaces, such as gingiva and the GI tract. Patients also often have multiple ecchymoses, and, of course, the platelet count is very low. The initial treatment involves trying to stop the autoimmune reaction, and this is best accomplished with prednisone. Most patients show a good response.

B. Although IVIg is used for refractory cases of ITP (where prednisone fails), it shouldn't be used as the first-line treatment.

C. Desmopressin is an analog of vasopressin, and used to treat von Willebrand's disease. This patient doesn't have this disease, which is characterized by prolonged bleeding time and prolonged PTT, but normal platelet count.

D. Vitamin K injection is usually used for prolonged PTT caused by vitamin K deficiency or to reverse Coumadin anticoagulation.

E. Protamine sulfate is used to reverse heparin anticoagulation.

133. D This set of markers represents an acute hepatitis B infection. Hepatitis B surface antigen is present whenever there is an active infection, either acute or chronic. Hepatitis B antigen represents a state of high infectivity, and thus would be present in the acute state. The first antibodies to appear in hepatitis B infection are those against the core antigen, with IgM antibodies appearing about six weeks after infection and IgG antibodies occurring about five to six months after infection. In this acute infection, there would be only IgM against the core antigen, as the IgG has not yet had to time to develop. The antibody to the surface antigen represents a state of immunity. In this active infection, it would not be present yet. If this patient goes on to have resolution, the anti-HBsAg would appear about six months after infection.

A. This set represents a patient who has been immunized by the HBV vaccine. He has antibody against the surface antigen and no detectable levels of any antigen.
B. This set represents a patient who has recovered from HBV infection and is now immune.
C. These are the markers that would be seen in someone who has a chronic infection with high infectivity. We know it is chronic by the presence of an IgG antibody against the core Ag (rather than IgM). We know it is unresolved because the anti-HBsAg is negative and the surface Ag is still present. It is classified as high infectivity because the e antigen is present. If the antibody to e antigen were measured, it would be negative.
E. This set is from someone who has chronic infection with low infectivity. It is similar to choice C, except the e antigen is not present, and anti-HBeAg would be negative.

134. C The patient has cystic fibrosis (CF), which is characterized by chronic airway infections, pancreatic insufficiency, intestinal obstruction, and failure to thrive. CF is an autosomal recessive disease resulting from mutations in a gene on chromosome 7. This gene encodes a protein known as the CF transmembrane regulator (CFTR). CFTR functions as a chloride ion channel and regulator of other ion channels.

A. Deficient phenylalanine hydroxylase is present in phenylketonuria (PKU), a disease characterized by mental retardation, fair skin, and eczema.
B. Lactase deficiency causes cramps, bloating, and diarrhea following ingestion of milk or milk products.
D. Potassium ion channels are normal in CF.

135. C Patterns of reinforcement (part of operant conditioning based on B.F. Skinner's work) include continuous, fixed, and variable. Variable reinforcement is the most difficult to extinguish; a classic example is why individuals continue to gamble when payoffs are so random and unpredictable, yet become outraged when a vending machine fails to produce a candy bar after money was deposited.

A. Continuous reinforcement involves a reward being presented after every target behavior; it is the easiest to extinguish.
B. Modeling is a form of observational learning in which actions of someone looked up to or admired are adopted.
D. Fixed reinforcement is presented after a certain fixed number of target behaviors (every third behavior is rewarded).
E. Variable reinforcement is more difficult to extinguish.

136. B ACE inhibitors have been found to be protective of the kidneys in several diseases including diabetes mellitus. Some clinicians would not use them if the creatinine is above 1.4 or 1.5. ACE inhibitors work to reduce hypertension by reducing the conversion of angiotensin I to angiotensin II in the lungs. Details of the protective effect on the kidneys are not known. Common side effects are cough, hyperkalemia, and rash. Other side effects include neutropenia and angioedema. ACE inhibitors are contraindicated in bilateral renal artery stenosis.

A. Beta-blockers may be dangerous in diabetes mellitus patients because they may block symptoms of hypoglycemia.
C. Alpha-blockers have not been shown to be protective in DM-II.
D. Too much diuresis may reduce blood flow to the kidneys causing acute rental failure.
E. Most calcium channel blockers are cleared by the kidneys, so should be used with caution in patients with impaired kidney function. They have not been shown to be of special benefit to diabetes mellitus patients.

137. E Based only on the history of what this patient told you, this patient has acquired *Histoplasma capsulatum*. This particular fungus is found in soil that is enriched with bird or bat feces. Since this patient did a lot of cave explorations, he most likely came in contact with this fungus without even realizing it. Microscopy reveals hyphae with microconidia and tuberculate macroconidia.

A. Primary TB has no environmental reservoirs even though the symptoms are similar to histoplasmosis. The x-ray would also be similar, however if we look closely at the patient's history it does not fit the profile.

B. Secondary TB is more extensive. It can be a multisystem disease not limiting itself to just the lungs. More lesions would be seen on x-ray.

C. *Blastomyces dermatitidis* is a form of fungus that is endemic to the Mississippi River, associated with rotting wood and beaver dams. The hotbeds of *Blastomyces* are located mainly in the Carolinas. Hyphae with nondescriptive conidia are seen under the microscope.

D. *Aspergillus fumigatus* is a fungus that is associated with those that work with compost pits and moldy marijuana. It can present as an allergic bronchopulmonary symptom. Monomorphic filamentous fungus with dichotomous branching is seen with the microscope.

138. A G6PD deficiency is an X-linked disorder affecting many individuals of African and Mediterranean descent. This disease is generally asymptomatic. However, during times of stress or exposure to oxidant drugs (such as sulfa and malaria drugs), hemolytic anemia results. G6PD deficiency affects more than 200 million people worldwide.

B. Pyruvate kinase deficiency results in a more severe hemolytic anemia that usually presents at a younger age.

C and D are incorrect, as deficiencies of these enzymes of glycolysis are extremely rare and would present with hemolytic anemia at a younger age.

139. A Based on the Social Readjustment Rating Scale from Holmes in 1978, psychosocial stressors are ranked according to the level of readjustment that will likely follow. The severity of these stressors is represented on Axis IV in the axial classification scheme for psychiatry based on the DSM. The most severe is death of spouse (with a mean value of 100) followed by divorce in the 70s.

B. Serious medical illness is ranked as more severe than change in residence.

C. Spouse's death is most severe, followed next by marriage, then birth of child.

D. Marital separation is most severe of these stressors.

E. Detention in jail requires only slightly less readjustment than separation, whereas trouble with boss is much lower on the scale.

140. B Psammoma bodies can be found in papillary carcinomas as well as meningiomas, mesotheliomas, and papillary cystadenoma of the ovaries. Papillary carcinomas are associated with previous exposure to ionizing radiation.

A. Papillary carcinoma is the most common form of thyroid cancer. Follicular carcinoma presents in older people as compared to papillary carcinoma. Follicular carcinoma is increased in areas of iodine deficiency and usually presents as a cold nodule.

C. It is true that medullary carcinomas are derived from C cells and it some cases they may release VIP. But they are not associated with MEN-I. Medullary carcinoma of thyroid is associated with MEN-III (type IIb).

D. Anaplastic carcinoma occurs mainly in older patients. The microscopic appearance is similar to small cell carcinoma.

141. B The cardiac cycle describes the sequential depolarization and re-polarization of the atrial and ventricular myocardium that leads (via excitation-contraction coupling) to the sequential contraction and relaxation of the atria and ventricles.

A. During isometric relaxation, ventricular volume remains the same. As the ventricular pressure decreases below the pressure of the atria, the mitral and tricuspid valves open and ventricular filling begins.

C. Incorrect.

D. Incorrect. As the aortic valve closes, the isometric relaxation period begins, and the blood volume in the ventricles at the beginning of isometric relaxation is equal to the end systolic volume.

E. Incorrect.

142. A Aspirin does not have an "antidote." The treatment for aspirin overdose is really only supportive, with close monitoring of fluids and electrolytes as well as acid-base balance. However, for acetaminophen overdosage, you need to protect the liver by providing acetylcysteine as glutathione is depleted. The therapeutic window for acetaminophen is quite large though. The usual dosage is 0.5 gm while hepatic toxic dosage is above 15 gm.

B. Dimercaprol is used in arsenic and mercury poisonings.

C. Naloxone is an antidote for opioids such as heroin.

D. Penicillamine is a chelating agent that is used to remove copper in Wilson's disease.

E. Deferoxamine is a chelating agent that binds with iron and is used in acute iron poisonings and in patients with chronic iron overload due to transfusion dependent anemias.

143. A A flagellate protozoan that causes steatorrhea due to malabsorption of fat from the duodenum and jejunum. It is primarily passed on through fecal-oral contamination commonly from drinking contaminated water.

B. Causes a bloody diarrhea. It produces flask-shaped ulcerations in the bowel and may produce amebic liver abscess.

C. Causes a transient diarrhea with acid-fast oocysts in the stool in healthy people. In the immunocompromised such as those with AIDS it can be intractable and life threatening.

D. *Trichomonas* produces a malodorous discharge coming from the vaginal vault in females. There is no diarrhea with this protozoan.

E. Not usually associated with disease in humans.

144. A Fabry's disease is a member of a group of diseases known as the lipid storage diseases. Fabry's disease is the result of an α-galactosidase deficiency. As a result, the body is unable to metabolize trihexosylceramide. Clinically, the patients present with a lower extremity rash, corneal opacities, fevers, and pain in the lower extremities. Death ensues secondary to renal and cardiac failure. Since the disease is X-linked recessive, the patient's sister is not homozygous but does have a mild variant of the disease, which resulted in the corneal opacities.

B. A deficiency in α-hexosaminidase A causes Tay-Sachs disease, which is characterized by mental retardation, the "cherry-red" spot on ophthalmic exam, weakness, and death, in the infantile form, by age 3 or 4.

C. A deficiency in α-glucosidase causes Gaucher's disease, which is characterized by mental retardation, hepatomegaly, splenomegaly, osteoporosis, and early death.

D. A deficiency in β-galactosidase causes Krabbe's disease, which is characterized by mental retardation, blindness, paralysis, and early death.

E. A deficiency in α-hexosaminidase A and B causes Sandhoff's disease which is characterized by mental retardation, the "cherry-red" spot on ophthalmic exam, weakness, and organomegaly.

145. D Diagnosis of posttraumatic stress disorder (PTSD) has four core elements—exposure to a traumatic event (the accident), re-experience of the event (nightmares and flashbacks), avoidance of triggers that are associated with the event (now afraid to drive), and new symptoms of increased arousal following the event (poor sleep, decreased concentration, irritability). Symptoms must last for at least one month and cause impairment in the individual's life.

A. Specific phobias are excessive or unreasonable fears brought on by the presence of a specific object or being. The individual is able to see that the fear is excessive.

B. Malingering is the conscious faking of a disorder in order to obtain a specific gain. Although always a consideration when accidents or legal claims are at stake, it wouldn't be highest on your differential at this point.

C. Dissociative disorder involves a break in the coordination of consciousness, memory, identity, or perception. Fugue is characterized by sudden inability to recall one's past and confusion about personal identity that accompanies sudden unexpected travel.

E. Given the duration and severity of symptoms, this is more than a normal reaction.

146. B The most prevalent organism affecting the lungs in patients with long-standing cystic fibrosis is *Pseudomonas aeruginosa*. The existence of a milder form of cystic fibrosis without the pancreatic insufficiency signs and symptoms is not unusual and can often be overlooked in patients with other medical problems such as psychiatric illness. With respect to the cephalosporins, cefepime, an "extended spectrum" third generation cephalosporin (sometimes called a fourth generation), provides the best coverage against *P. aeruginosa*.

A. Cefoxitin is a second generation cephalosporin with anaerobic coverage and is good for colorectal surgery prophylaxis, intra-abdominal infections, aspiration pneumonias, and pelvic inflammatory disease

C. Cefixime is a third generation cephalosporin. These cover hospital-acquired (nosocomial) pneumonia, meningitis, sepsis, and UTIs. They also cover multidrug resistant aerobic gram-negative organisms, and are the preferred coverage for *Klebsiella* pneumonia. Cefixime provides no coverage of infections due to *P. aeruginosa*.

D. Ceftriaxone is a third generation cephalosporin like cefixime and is the prototype drug. It has no coverage for *P. aeruginosa*. In addition, it has the longest half life of all cephalosporins and has the best CSF penetration for use in meningitis. It is excreted in bile, so it can be used in renal failure patients. It also has excellent bone penetration. Lastly, it is often used to treat *Neisseria gonorrhoeae*.

E. Cefaclor is not effective against *Pseudomonas*.

147. E Defense mechanisms are methods used by the ego to handle psychological stress. Regression is characterized by returning to behavior patterns as seen in someone younger.

A. Sublimation is characterized by replacing unacceptable feelings into a socially acceptable action.

B. Denial is characterized by not believing in a reality because it is too painful.

C. Suppression is characterized by consciously pushing away a thought or emotion from awareness.

D. Repression is characterized by unconsciously pushing away a thought or emotion from awareness.

148. D TB is caused by *Mycobacterium tuberculosis* (sometimes called tubercle bacillus). It is an acid-fast bacilli that is intracellular, grows slowly, and acquires rapid resistance to drug therapy. TB is the number one cause of death from infectious disease worldwide. TB cases continue to be reported all across the United States. In 1998, a total of 18,361 new cases (rate of 6.8/100,000) of TB were reported to the CDC. Although nonspecific, a posterior-anterior plain chest film is the most commonly used imaging tool for detecting tuberculosis. The lung lesions are usually located in the apical and posterior upper lobe lung segments or in the superior segments of the lower lobe. Pulmonary TB symptoms include cough, chest pain, and hemoptysis. Systemic systems consistent

with TB include fever, chills, night sweats, appetite loss, weight loss, and fatigability. A complete medical evaluation for TB includes a medical history, a physical examination, a Mantoux tuberculin skin test, a chest radiograph, and any appropriate bacteriologic/histologic examinations. Isoniazid (INH) is a key agent in the treatment of *M. tuberculosis*. It is a bactericidal drug that interferes with the mycolic acid component in the cell wall of the mycobacterium. INH increases the excretion of vitamin B_6 (pyridoxine), a water soluble vitamin, causing vitamin B_6 deficiency and subsequent triad of pellagra—dementia, dermatitis, and diarrhea. These side effects can be reduced/reversed with the administration of vitamin B_6.

A. This is a fat-soluble vitamin that is administered in diseases that cause malabsorption problems. It is needed for bone development, growth, and adaptation to darkness.

B. This is a water-soluble vitamin commonly used in the treatment of pernicious anemia, hemorrhage, or to supplement the increased requirement during pregnancy.

C. This is a water-soluble vitamin used to prevent scurvy and help acidify the urine during drug toxicities.

E. This is a fat-soluble vitamin used as a dietary supplement with an antioxidant scavenging component.

149. D This patient is experiencing hemorrhagic shock from placenta previa. Shock is a state of inadequate tissue perfusion. The best initial tool for measuring adequacy of tissue perfusion is checking the patient's level of consciousness, which is indicative of brain perfusion. The brain is the most sensitive organ to shock.

A. Metabolic acidosis is a result of inadequate tissue perfusion.

B. Although carbon dioxide will increase in an inverse relationship to pH, reflecting the metabolic acidotic state, this is an effect of inadequate tissue perfusion.

C. Cells become more permeable during a breakdown of the oxidative chain pathway and a failure to maintain cell structure. Waste by-products from anaerobic metabolism leak out and contribute to the metabolic acidosis.

E. Urinary output is a sensitive measurement of adequacy of kidney perfusion during shock states, and blood glucose levels increase during any stress placed on the body. However, these are the effects of inadequate tissue perfusion.

150. B The joint aspirate shows the typical needle-shaped, negatively birefringent crystals of uric acid. This patient is suffering from an acute attack of gout. Indomethacin is the NSAID of choice for acute gouty arthritis. A high dose and short course are used to decrease possible complications from the medicines. One possible regimen is indomethacin 50 mg three to four times a day for three to five days.

A. Medicines like allopurinol (Zyloprim) are inhibitors of uric acid production but are not used in acute gout. These medicines can cause an initial increase of uric acid.

C. This class of medicines is used in chronic gout but less frequently. They are known to inhibit the renal tubular resorption of uric acid, thus decreasing uric acid concentrations in the blood.

D. Not all the NSAIDs are indicated in acute gout! Aspirin has been shown to cause a worsening of symptoms and may actually exacerbate the arthritis.

E. Naproxen and diclofenac are NSAIDs often used other than indomethacin. The COX-II inhibitors can be used in patients who cannot tolerate other NSAIDs.

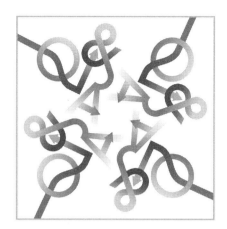

QUESTIONS
BLOCK 4

151. A 50-year-old male alcoholic presents to the ER with epigastric abdominal pain radiating to his back, nausea, vomiting, and a low-grade fever. He states that this has happened two times before and that it is always an acute-onset event. The pain is relieved by sitting up and leaning forward. Serum amylase and lipase are markedly elevated. Which of the following best applies to this disorder?

   A. Pseudocysts are a rare and benign complication.

   B. Alcohol and gallstones are the etiologic factor in less than 50% of cases in the United States.

   C. Increased levels of amylase are a less specific marker than increased levels of lipase.

   D. A strong correlation between this disorder and pancreatic cancer has been noted.

   E. Trypsin, synthesized in its active form, is the enzyme that activates various proenzymes and thus autodigestion.

152. A couple complains that they have had difficulty conceiving. Physical examination and basic laboratory tests are within normal limits. What drug regimen would you suggest?

   A. Clomiphene

   B. Tamoxifen

   C. Mifepristone

   D. Levonorgestrel

   E. Medroxyprogesterone

153. A 30-year-old male business executive comes to your office with a two-day complaint of fever, general malaise, productive cough, sore throat, and postnasal drainage. The patient has otherwise been healthy with no significant medical history. You suspect the patient has a viral respiratory infection and treat appropriately. With respect to the respiratory disease process described in this patient, the central chemoreceptors responsible for triggering respirations are directly stimulated by:

   A. Decrease in $PaCO_2$

   B. Increase in $PaCO_2$

   C. Decrease in serum pH

   D. Decrease in PaO_2

   E. Increase in PaO_2

154. A woman brings her 3-year-old son into the pediatrician's office because she noticed a "bulge in his belly." Exam reveals a hernia in the inguinal region. During surgery it is noted that this hernia is lateral to the inferior epigastric vessels. **(See Figure 154.)** Which of the following applies best to this hernia?

   A. It passes through Hesselbach's triangle.

   B. The hernia sac does not pass through the deep inguinal ring.

   C. The hernia sac represents the remains of the processus vaginalis.

   D. It frequently results from weakening of the conjoint tendon.

   E. This hernia is the most common hernia in males but not females.

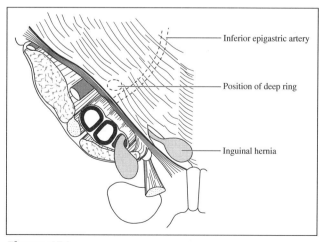

Figure 154

155. The roommate of a 19-year-old male is concerned about his recent odd behavior. Six months prior he began withdrawing from his friends and stopped going to classes. He also would occasionally burst out laughing in the middle of serious conversations and walk away mumbling to himself. Today he barricaded himself in his room, refusing to come out, and is ranting about the CIA spying on him through cracks in the walls and with look-a-like impostors.

Regarding the treatment options for this illness:

- **A.** Typical antipsychotics treat the negative symptoms with greater efficacy than the positive symptoms.
- **B.** The family of atypical antipsychotics bears no resemblance to each other in terms of chemical formula.
- **C.** With proper management the patient will most likely regain his pre-illness level of social functioning.
- **D.** Family and social support does not play an integral role in the patient's treatment program.
- **E.** Parkinsonian-type symptoms are associated with the atypical antipsychotics.

156. An 18-year-old woman with a history of asthma presents to your clinic with shortness of breath and expiratory wheezing. You decide to treat her with inhaled albuterol and a course of prednisone. The albuterol produces an almost immediate improvement in her symptoms, while prednisone will take several hours to have its maximal benefit. Which of the following explains why prednisone and other steroid hormones take several hours to exert their effect?

- **A.** It acts on cytoplasmic receptors, leading to enhanced transcription of specific genes.
- **B.** It acts on cell surface receptors, initiating a variety of signalization cascades.
- **C.** It binds directly to DNA to enhance the transcription of specific genes.
- **D.** It prevents degradation of specific types of mRNA in the cytoplasm.

157. Your college roommate is complaining of headache and fever. The following day you try to arouse him from bed and are not able to do so. He is immediately taken to the emergency room. CBC showed a WBC of 21,000 with 90% PMNs. Cerebrospinal fluid was cloudy. Analysis of the CSF showed 1000 PMNs/ mm^3, glucose of 2 mg/dl, and protein of 110 mg/dl. What should the physician suspect?

- **A.** Gram-negative diplococcus species
- **B.** Gram-positive coccus, catalase negative, and gamma hemolytic

- **C.** Gram-positive coccus, catalase positive, and bacitracin resistant
- **D.** Western equine encephalitis
- **E.** Measles virus

158. An infectious disease specialist relates to you that there is a new mutant species of a pathogenic bacteria. This mutant differs in that there are changes involving the 30s ribosome subunit, which may lead to resistance to some antibiotics. If a patient came in affected with this mutant strain, which antibiotic would still most likely be effective?

- **A.** Tetracycline
- **B.** Spectinomycin
- **C.** Amikacin
- **D.** Gentamicin
- **E.** Chloramphenicol

159. A 59-year-old man presents with a six-month history of cough, dyspnea, hemoptysis, weight loss, and fatigue. Recently, he complains that his left eyelid is drooping. He has difficulty seeing from the left eye and noticed an absence of sweating on the face. He has a history of treated tuberculosis and a 36 pack-per-year history of smoking, but he quit smoking when these symptoms began. A chest x-ray shows a 5-cm mass localized in the left apical lung with invasion to the cervical region. Ptosis of the left eyelid is most likely caused by damage to what nerve?

- **A.** CN III
- **B.** CN IV
- **C.** CN VI
- **D.** Sympathetic nerve
- **E.** CN II

160. The parents of an 18-month-old boy are concerned because he frequently becomes hyperpneic, turns blue, and then passes out during crying episodes. There is a systolic murmur heard best at the left sternal border, and EKG shows right axis deviation and an RSR pattern. Echocardiogram confirms the suspicion of tetralogy of Fallot. **(See Figure 160.)** The most likely shunt pattern and myocardial change associated with this will be:

- **A.** Right to left shunt, right ventricular hypertrophy
- **B.** Left to right shunt, right ventricular hypertrophy
- **C.** Left to right shunt, left ventricular hypertrophy
- **D.** Right to left shunt, left ventricular hypertrophy
- **E.** No shunt, biventricular hypertrophy

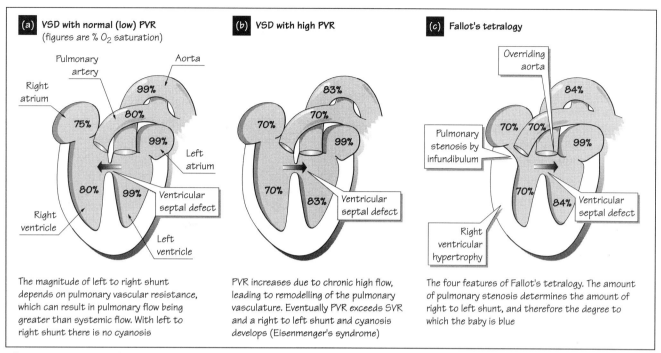

(a) VSD with normal (low) PVR
(figures are % O_2 saturation)

The magnitude of left to right shunt depends on pulmonary vascular resistance, which can result in pulmonary flow being greater than systemic flow. With left to right shunt there is no cyanosis

(b) VSD with high PVR

PVR increases due to chronic high flow, leading to remodelling of the pulmonary vasculature. Eventually PVR exceeds SVR and a right to left shunt and cyanosis develops (Eisenmenger's syndrome)

(c) Fallot's tetralogy

The four features of Fallot's tetralogy. The amount of pulmonary stenosis determines the amount of right to left shunt, and therefore the degree to which the baby is blue

Figure 160   Reproduced with permission from Aaronson. The Cardiovascular System at a Glance. Blackwell Science, Ltd., 1999.

161. A 35-year-old female presents to her primary care physician's office for the third time this month. She is dressed very provocatively and is very preoccupied with her appearance. As with her two previous visits, the physician notes that he is unable to elicit a specific complaint from the patient. The patient makes frequent, sexually inappropriate comments toward the physician. She demands that the physician stay in the exam room with her, instead of seeing other patients. Which personality disorder is this patient displaying?

A. Antisocial

B. Schizoid

C. Histrionic

D. Avoidant

E. Dependent

162. While doing an emergency medicine rotation in the middle of winter, you respond with paramedics to a man with a headache. Inside you find an elderly man who heats his house with a kerosene heater. The patient is agitated, confused, and has two episodes of emesis while attending to him. You suspect carbon monoxide intoxication. The effects of carbon monoxide on the oxygen dissociation curve are shown in the graph. **(See Figure 162.)** Which curve binds oxygen with the greatest affinity?

A. Curve A

B. Curve B

C. Curve C

D. Curve D

E. Curve E

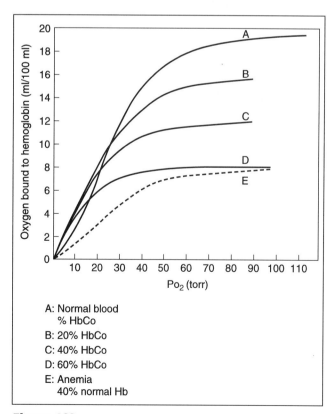

A: Normal blood
% HbCo
B: 20% HbCo
C: 40% HbCo
D: 60% HbCo
E: Anemia
40% normal Hb

Figure 162

163. A 45-year-old white male comes to your office with a painful swollen foot. He has had diabetes mellitus type I for 28 years. He is on insulin, but otherwise takes no medications and has no allergies. Upon exam of the foot, you notice an abscess and incise it. The draining fluid has a faint blue-green coloring to it and smells like sweet grape juice. A quick Gram's stain shows gram-negative rods. The most likely organism based on this description and history is:

A. *Staphylococcus aureus*

B. *Proteus vulgaris*

C. *Clostridium perfringens*

D. *Streptococcus pyogenes*

E. *Pseudomonas aeruginosa*

164. A 65-year-old black man is referred to your office for treatment of essential hypertension. He relates that his only other medical problem is that he has severe osteoarthritis in his left knee for which he frequently takes aspirin. In considering a medicine to manage his hypertension, which agent should be eliminated from consideration as a first line agent?

A. Furosemide

B. Nifedipine

C. Methyldopa

D. Clonidine

E. Lisinopril

165. A 35-year-old male presents with a history of increasing difficulty with choreiform movements, emotional lability, and symptoms suggestive of dementia. His father had a similar condition and died at a relatively young age. Which of the following correctly pairs the disease process with its associated neurotransmitter abnormality?

A. Huntington's disease/decreased GABA

B. Schizophrenia/decreased dopamine

C. Parkinson's disease/increased dopamine

D. Alzheimer's dementia/increased acetylcholine

E. Depression/increased serotonin

166. A 60-year-old man is found on a routine physical to have bilaterally nonreactive pupils. The pupils do, however, accommodate for near vision. The patient recalls an episode years ago of palm and foot rashes accompanied by fever. What organism is most likely the cause of his pupillary findings?

A. *Mycobacterium tuberculosis*

B. *Borrelia burgdorferi*

C. *Legionella pneumophila*

D. *Francisella tularensis*

E. *Treponema pallidum*

167. A 30-year-old female was brought to the emergency room with a four-day history of severe vomiting. Her blood pressure was 90/50 mm Hg, respiratory rate was 14 breaths per minute, and she displayed poor tissue turgor. She was given IV fluids and several labs were drawn. The following are her arterial blood values:

pH   = 7.60

pCO_2 = 55 mm Hg

$[HCO_3^-]$ = 63 mEq/L

Venous blood samples show decreased blood $[K^+]$ and $[Cl^-]$ levels. The correct diagnosis for this patient is:

A. Respiratory alkalosis

B. Metabolic alkalosis with respiratory compensation

C. Respiratory acidosis

D. Metabolic acidosis with respiratory compensation

E. Normal acid-base status

168. A 43-year-old female with a history of anxiety is brought to the emergency department via ambulance. Paramedics report that the patient was found unresponsive at home by her husband. On arrival, the patient is bradycardic and hypotensive, with a decreased respiratory rate. The patient arouses to painful stimuli, but is only oriented to self. On further exam, the patient is found to have decreased deep tendon reflexes. The physician suspects that the patient has overdosed on benzodiazepines. What medication can be given to try to reverse the effects of benzodiazepines?

A. Naloxone

B. Edetate

C. Deferoxamine

D. Flumazenil

E. Acetylcysteine

169. A 35-year-old woman presents with a cervical carcinoma. Which of the following viruses is associated with cervical carcinoma?

A. Human Papillomavirus 1 (HPV-1)

B. Human Papillomavirus 6 (HPV-6)

C. Human Papillomavirus 11 (HPV-11)

D. Human Papillomavirus 16 (HPV-16)

E. Epstein-Barr virus (EBV)

170. A 50-year-old homeless man is brought to the emergency room acutely intoxicated. On examination, you observe bleeding from gums and extensive bruising. You suspect the diagnosis of scurvy due to lack of dietary vitamin C. Which of the following proteins is produced abnormally in this disease?

A. Insulin

B. Coagulation factors II, VII, IX, and X

C. Globin

D. Collagen

171. A 23-year-old medical student presents to the emergency department following a disturbing experience that has occurred now twice in the past week. She describes that prior to and during her first two exams of medical school she had acute onset of palpitations, sweating, nausea, and overwhelming worry that she would fail her test. The first occurred during an anatomy lab practical, and she was not able to finish the exam. The second occurred during a sit-down physiology exam which she was not able to finish. She is now very fearful that she will not be able to perform up to her ability. She is very invested in getting this figured out, stating it has always been her goal to become a doctor. You suspect which of the following?

A. Specific phobia

B. Viral illness

C. Malingering

D. Formaldehyde allergy

E. Panic attack

172. A 54 year-old comes into the emergency room complaining of fatigue. He is breathing at 30 breaths per minute and says he is getting tired. An ABG and SMA-7 are done and show the following results **(Table 172)**:

When asked about past medical history, the patient states he was diagnosed with type II diabetes mellitus six years ago. He has been taking medicine for it, but doesn't know which one. Which medication is this patient most likely taking?

A. Glyburide

B. Rosiglitazone

C. Insulin

D. Acarbose

E. Metformin

Table 172

ABG		SMA-7	
pH	7.30	Na	139 mEq/L
pCO$_2$	34 mm Hg	K	4.9 mEq/L
pO$_2$	99 mm Hg	Cl	100 mEq/L
HCO$_3$	16 mEq/L	HCO$_3$	16 mEq/L
O$_2$ sat	99%	BUN	22 mg/dL
		Cr	1.4 mg/dL
		Glucose	146 mg/dL

173. A 45-year-old male presents to the emergency room complaining of headaches, dizziness, and fatigue. He has recently been diagnosed with essential hypertension and was started on a diuretic by his primary care physician. Labs reveal that the patient is hyponatremic, hypokalemic, hypercalcemic, and has an elevated blood pH. Which is the most likely diuretic the patient is taking?

A. Spironolactone

B. Furosemide

C. Hydrochlorothiazide

D. Triamterene

E. Ethacrynic acid

174. A 27-year-old male patient presents three weeks status post gunshot wound to the thigh entering approximately halfway between the hip and knee. The metal-cased bullet entered the lateral thigh and exited the medial thigh. The patient presents with weakness of the leg. If the sciatic nerve were severed, which of the following muscles would likely be normal by EMG studies? **(See Figure 174.)**

A. Gastrocnemius

B. Biceps femoris

C. Tibialis anterior

D. Vastus medialis

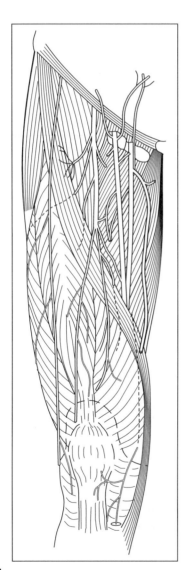

Figure 174

175. A 33-year-old male is brought to the emergency department unconscious. Blood chemistries are drawn, a lumbar puncture done, and a history taken from a friend that indicates that the patient had been very despondent. Which of the following CSF findings has been associated with a high rate of suicide completion?

A. Increased protein

B. Presence of red blood cells

C. Decreased 5-HIAA

D. Increased 5-HIAA

E. Decreased glucose

176. A culture flask is one-eighth filled with *E. coli*, a bacteria that has a generation time of 20 minutes. How long will it take before the flask is filled?

A. 20 minutes

B. 40 minutes

C. 1 hour

D. 2 hours

E. 4 hours

177. When it comes to older patients, which of the following holds true?

A. Polypharmacy, OTC medications, increased body size, increased body water, increased body fat, decreased phase 1 reaction, decreased renal flow

B. Polypharmacy, OTC medications, decreased body size, decreased body water, decreased body fat, decreased phase 1 reaction, decreased renal flow

C. Polypharmacy, OTC medications, increased body size, increased body water, increased body fat, decreased phase 1 reaction, decreased renal flow

D. Polypharmacy, OTC medications, decreased body size, decreased body water, decreased body fat, decreased phase 1 reaction, decreased renal flow

E. Polypharmacy, OTC medications, decreased body size, decreased body water, increased body fat, decreased phase 1 reaction, decreased renal flow

178. A 25-year-old man presented to the ER with an acute onset of coughing up blood and shortness of breath. On physical exam, he is afebrile and has chest retractions with decreased breath sounds. He also has hematuria. What is most likely seen on renal biopsy using immunofluorescence?

A. Granular pattern

B. Crescent-moon shape

C. Mesangial deposits of IgA

D. Linear pattern of antiglobular basement membrane antibodies

179. A 68-year-old woman presents to your office complaining of burning, frequency, and urgency of urination. Urinalysis reveals many white blood cells, and urine cultures grow colonies of *E. coli* that are resistant to ciprofloxacin, a fluoro-quinolone antibiotic. What is a potential genetic mechanism of resistance in these bacteria?

A. Production of β-lactamase

B. Altered methylation of 50S ribosomal subunit

C. Altered methylation of 30S ribosomal subunit

D. Mutation of gene encoding DNA gyrase

180. A 65-year-old white male comes to the office. He has recently had abdominal surgery, and the chart note written by your assistant says he fell down today. You are about to begin taking a history from him. Which of the following would be considered an open-ended question?

A. On a scale of one to 10, where do you rate your pain today?

B. What happened when you fell down today?

C. Have you passed gas since your surgery?

D. Are your relatives out in the waiting room?

E. This must be difficult for you. Would you like to take a break?

181. A 73-year-old man presents with intermittent chest discomfort. A diagnostic cardiac catheterization reveals diffuse disease of the left anterior descending (LAD) coronary artery. The diameter of the artery has been reduced to one-half of its original size (50% occlusion). The flow of blood in this artery has been decreased to what proportion of its original blood flow?

A. One-half (50%)

B. One-fourth (25%)

C. One-eighth (12.5%)

D. 1/16 (6.3%)

E. 1/64 (3.1%)

182. You have a patient diagnosed with diabetes insipidus with a nephrogenic origin. Which of the following drugs would be most useful?

A. Lypressin

B. Vasopressin

C. Thiazides

D. Desmopressin

183. A 31-year-old nulliparous woman comes to your office complaining of one week of minor burning and itching of her labia. She also states that she has excessive vaginal discharge that is foul-smelling. The patient has no abnormalities of menstruation and is currently midcycle. She is sexually active and in a monogamous relationship. You do a full pelvic exam and collect vaginal discharge for examination under the microscope. The slide shows vaginal epithelial cells with dozens of small dots within the cells. **(See Figure 183.)** The most likely cause of this woman's vaginitis is:

A. *Candida albicans*

B. *Trichomonas vaginalis*

C. *Gardnerella vaginalis*

D. *Neisseria gonorrhoeae*

E. *Chlamydia trachomatis*

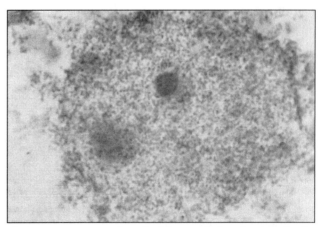

Figure 183 Reproduced with permission from Axford. Medicine. Blackwell Science, Ltd., 1996.

184. Late one night on the wards, the intern asks you to put a central line in the left femoral vein of a patient. After a successful procedure, the nurse calls you and says that the patient is having pain in his groin. On exam, you discover a painful, bluish mass at the site of line insertion. Which of the following is consistent with this finding?

A. Increased hematocrit

B. Hypertension

C. Decreased peripheral pulse in the left foot

D. Warm left foot

185. An 18-year-old Caucasian male arrives in the emergency room complaining of "bugs crawling all over me." Otherwise, the patient appears euphoric. His vitals reveal a heart rate of 120 and a blood pressure of 160/100 mm Hg. On physical exam, you note pupils are dilated. Throughout the exam, he is brushing off imaginary bugs from his body. What substance has this patient most likely taken?

A. He is withdrawing from a heroin injection.

B. He has taken cocaine within the hour.

C. He is withdrawing from amphetamines.

D. He has smoked PCP within the hour.

E. He has ingested LSD within the hour.

186. A 42-year-old man presents to your office for a routine physical examination and screening tests. Laboratory testing reveals a total cholesterol level of 300 mg/dL and LDL cholesterol of 210 mg/dL. Treatment with lovastatin is initiated. Lovastatin has which of the following primary mechanisms of action?

A. Decreases the reabsorption of bile acids in the intestine

B. Decreases the biosynthesis of cholesterol in hepatocytes

C. Reduces fat absorption through inhibition of gastric and pancreatic lipase

D. Increases the activity of lipoprotein lipase (LPL)

187. An 85-year-old man presents to your office because of recurrent fainting. The fainting has occurred on three occasions when the patient stood up quickly. On these occasions he feels lightheaded and describes darkness closing in on his vision prior to losing consciousness. He has not been confused or had any neurological deficit following these episodes of fainting. On several other occasions, he has suffered severe lightheadedness on standing that is relieved by sitting back down. He reports good intake of fluids and denies vomiting, diarrhea, or bleeding. However, he suffers from long-standing, poorly controlled diabetes mellitus and decreased sensation in his lower extremities bilaterally. Which of the following is likely responsible for his fainting?

A. Autonomic insufficiency

B. Diffuse sensory neuropathy

C. Cerebrovascular accident

D. Peripheral vascular disease

188. A 38-year-old male patient, who had a long-time history of IV drug abuse with needle sharing, comes to the emergency department after having severe attacks of pain. The patient describes an intense, sharp, stabbing, right-sided flank pain that is intermittent but frequent. The patient's urine dipstick is positive for blood. You have been treating this patient for more than five months and now on physical examination in the ED you notice continued spread of multiple endothelial cell tumors over his chest and abdomen. You also observe a peculiar adipose tissue redistribution with loss of facial fat, increased internal abdominal fat accumulation, and dorsocervical tissue accumulation. These metabolic side effects are most likely due to?

A. Zidovudine

B. Zalcitabine

C. Abacavir

D. Efavirenz

E. Indinavir

189. Mrs. Martin is a 70-year-old retired schoolteacher. Her daughter is concerned about her mother's gradually increasing forgetfulness. During the history and physical exam, you determine that the most likely cause for the cognitive impairment is normal pressure hydrocephalus. Which clue led you to that conclusion?

A. Recent weight gain

B. Recent head trauma

C. Handwriting smaller than usual

D. Forgetting to turn off the stove

E. Gait ataxia, forgetfulness, and urinary incontinence

F. Urinary incontinence and recent head trauma

190. A 23-year-old Hispanic male comes into the outpatient clinic complaining of mild fever, severe sore throat, and swollen glands in his inguinal region three months prior to this visit. He saw a doctor, who told him he had the flu, and was given no medicine. He also states he has been feeling very fatigued for the last few weeks, but the other symptoms have resolved. His lymph nodes are still swollen. On history, the patient admits to shooting heroin and has had numerous sexual partners in the last year. He states that sometimes he uses condoms and sometimes he does not. You suspect possible HIV infection, and advise the patient that an HIV test should be done. He agrees and an ELISA test is performed, which comes back positive. A repeat HIV ELISA is still positive. What should be the next step in the management of this patient?

A. Order another ELISA test in one month.

B. Order a Western blot test.

C. Begin the patient on a cocktail of reverse transcriptase inhibitors.

D. Begin the patient on PCP prophylaxis with Bactrim.

E. Place the patient in isolation.

191. A 14-week-old infant who was the product of an uneventful full-term pregnancy suddenly became progressively lethargic, stopped feeding, and vomited. The infant was found to be dehydrated, with a serum sodium level of 128 mEq/L, and hypotensive. Further work-up revealed that the infant, thought to be a boy at birth by appearance of the external genitalia, had a 46 XX karyotype. Which of the following enzymes is most likely defective in this patient?

A. 21-alpha-hydroxylase

B. 11-beta-hydroxylase

C. 17-alpha-hydroxylase

D. Homogentisic oxidase

E. Alpha-L-iduronidase

192. A 20-year-old female presents to the office with a complaint of a severe headache. Which of the following questions is the best way to begin the patient interview?

A. Is the headache on one side or both sides?

B. Is the pain sharp or dull?

C. Tell me about your headache.

D. Are you hurting anywhere else besides your head?

E. How severe is the pain?

193. A 9-year-old male presents to your office. He has been treated for tonic-clonic seizures for the past six years. During his exam you notice that he has coarse facial features and gums that extend down over much of his teeth. The medication that he has been on is:

A. Phenytoin

B. Carbamazepine

C. Phenobarbital

D. Valproic acid

E. Clonazepam

194. You are part of the Flying Doctors of Mercy. They fly to third-world countries providing free health care. You have a patient with swollen gums, anemia, and history of poor wound healing. Which vitamin deficiency is causing these symptoms?

A. Vitamin A

B. Vitamin B_1

C. Vitamin B_2

D. Vitamin B_6

E. Vitamin C

F. Vitamin D

G. Vitamin E

195. A 25-year-old white male presents to the emergency department with weakness that initially started in his arms but has now spread throughout his body, double vision, and difficulty swallowing. He has not had any fever and denies any significant medical, surgical, and family history. About two days ago, he scratched his foot while walking on the beach. The area of scratch is slightly erythematous, but without drainage. Patient's blood culture had no bacterial growth but presence of a toxin of anaerobic gram-positive rod is found.

The treatment for the problem at hand is:

A. Supportive

B. Vaccine

C. Antitoxin

D. Debridement of the wound

E. IV antibiotics

196. A 31-year-old pregnant African-American female visits your clinic for the first time, having had no prenatal care. You determine by last menstrual period, physical exam, and ultrasound that she is about 20 weeks pregnant. She informs you that her husband has sickle cell disease, and her 8-year-old son is a carrier. She does not know her own genetic status, but knows that she has never had any symptoms of sickle cell disease. You obtain DNA samples from the fetus by amniocentesis, as well as from the mother and father. These samples are then amplified by PCR and then tested under stringent conditions using allele-specific oligonucleotide probes (ASO probes), one for the normal allele and one for the mutant allele of the beta-globin gene. Of the following dot blots **(see Figure 196)**, which one represents a possible result that could be obtained from this test on this family, given this limited information? (NP = ASO probe for normal allele, SP = ASO probe for mutant allele, M = mother, Fa = father, Fe = fetus.)

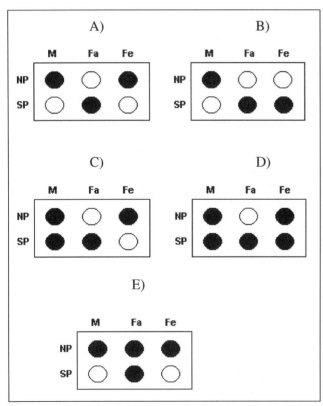

Figure 196

197. You are working for a pharmaceutical company and have been involved in the formulation of a new drug. One of the concerns is bioavailability. Bioavailability of this drug may be affected by:

A. First-pass hepatic metabolism

B. Solubility

C. Nature of drug formulation

D. Chemical instability

E. All of the above

198. A 73-year-old Hispanic gentleman visits your clinic in Phoenix, Arizona. He complains of persistent headache, fever, and neck pain for the past three days; these symptoms were preceded by two to three weeks of malaise, chest pain, and a persistent cough with sputum production. He also reveals a 10-pound weight loss in the past three weeks. Upon pulmonary examination, there is dullness to percussion over the right upper lung field, as well as increased tactile fremitus and bronchial breath sounds in this same region. You also notice deep, red nodules, very tender to palpation bilaterally on both lower extremities. A chest x-ray is consistent with your examination, though it also demonstrates hilar lymphadenopathy. CSF appears clear, pressure is 190 mm (NL 70–180), WBC 250 cells/uL (lymphocyte predominant), glucose 25 mg/dL (NL 40–70), protein 55 mg/dL (NL 15–45). Direct examination of a smear from CSF is negative for any organisms. Direct examination of sputum reveals nonbudding spherical forms full of endospores.

Which of the following is true concerning the organism responsible for this disease?

A. It exists in the environment as conidial molds, microconidia being the infectious form which is inhaled.

B. It is a facultative intracellular parasite, being found in reticuloendothelial cells.

C. Specimens obtained via bronchoalveolar lavage are necessary for a definitive diagnosis.

D. Disseminated disease has a tendency to develop in the third trimester of pregnancy.

E. HIV+ patients with CD4+ counts less than 200/uL should receive prophylactic treatment against this disease.

199. A 15-year-old girl states that since the age of 11, the girls in her class have made fun of her because she does not have her period and does not need or wear a bra. Today, she is nervous about the upcoming homecoming dance. She is complaining that whenever she wears a dress, it never looks right because her neck "sticks out." On exam, she is short, with a broad chest with wide spaced nipples, and unusually short fourth metacarpal. Which of the following genotypes is most consistent with the patient's history and physical?

A. 46, XX

B. 47, XY

C. 47, XY

D. 46, XO

E. 47, XXX

200. A 70-year-old African-American man with urinary retention and benign prostatic hyperplasia develops fever, chills, hypotension, and sinus tachycardia. He has a full pulse and warm and dry skin. His complete blood count shows absolute neutrophil count of 200. The hemodynamic findings in this patient are probably the result of:

A. Endotoxemia and complement system activation

B. Endothelial damage due to invasive bacteria penetrating the cells

C. Reflex vasodilation compensating for reduced cardiac output

D. Peripheral vasoconstriction resulting in high-output failure

E. Reflex sympathetic relaxation with reduction in cardiac output

BLOCK IV - ANSWER KEY

151-C	164-E	177-E	189-E
152-A	165-A	178-D	190-B
153-B	166-E	179-D	191-A
154-C	167-B	180-B	192-C
155-B	168-D	181-D	193-A
156-A	169-D	182-C	194-E
157-A	170-D	183-C	195-C
158-E	171-E	184-C	196-D
159-D	172-E	185-B	197-E
160-A	173-C	186-B	198-D
161-C	174-D	187-A	199-D
162-D	175-C	188-E	200-A
163-E	176-C		

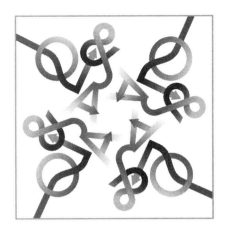

ANSWERS
BLOCK 4

151. C Other disorders, including perforated gastric ulcers, sialolithiasis, intestinal obstructions, or pancreatic cancer can all increase amylase. Lipase, however, is a far more specific marker. Used together, amylase and lipase measurements are both highly sensitive and specific for acute pancreatitis.

A. Pancreatic pseudocysts are quite common and can rupture, spilling pancreatic enzymes into the peritoneal cavity.
B. These two factors account for more than 80% of the cases in the United States.
D. The only known risk factor for pancreatic cancer is smoking.
E. Although trypsin activates the other enzymes, it is synthesized as a proenzyme. This is significant because this is the limiting step in the cascade leading to autodigestion.

152. A Clomiphene is a partial estrogen agonist that causes an increase in LH and FSH. It will stimulate ovulation and has been implicated in multiple births.

B. Tamoxifen is a selective estrogen receptor modulator working only in the breast, uterus, and bone. It is used as prophylaxis against breast cancer.
C. Mifepristone is better known as RU486. It is an antiprogestin and used to terminate pregnancy.
D. Levonorgestrel is a progestin implant that inhibits ovulation.
E. Medroxyprogesterone is a progestin that inhibits ovulation.

153. B The patient is a healthy individual with normal respiratory physiological processes who has an upper respiratory viral infection. This patient's respiratory drive is under the influence of central chemoreceptor cells located on the ventral surface of the brainstem. They are not the same cells that make up the medullary respiratory neurons. These central chemoreceptors stimulate breathing when $PaCO_2$ is elevated. These central chemoreceptors respond rapidly to changes in arterial $PaCO_2$ and the resultant changes in pH. Due to the blood-brain barrier H^+ ions are not able to cross and only CO_2 can cross, which is what the central chemoreceptors respond to. Respiration triggered by central chemoreceptors is not normally triggered by hypoxia. It is interesting to note that in chronic bronchitis (a form of COPD), patients retain high levels of CO_2 (blue bloaters) and their central chemoreceptors reset after prolonged exposure to high $PaCO_2$. When $PaCO_2$ rises too high, it acts as a narcotic and inactivates the central chemoreceptors. These COPD patients then have their respirations influenced by peripheral chemoreceptors that measure levels of PaO_2. When PaO_2 levels decrease, peripheral chemoreceptors stimulate respiration. This is known as hypoxic drive. Although not adequately proven, hypoxic drive COPD patients who are in respiratory distress theoretically may be placed into respiratory arrest by applying high-dose oxygen, since the peripheral chemoreceptors will not trigger respirations in the face of high PaO_2.

A. Only increases in $PaCO_2$ affect respirations.
C. Although a low pH will also be found, it is the CO_2 that can cross the blood-brain barrier, not the H^+ ions.
D. This works to stimulate breathing only in hypoxic drive patients.
E. High levels of oxygen do not trigger a healthy individual to breathe.

154. C The description given above describes an indirect inguinal hernia. The hernia sac represents the remains of the processus vaginalis, an evagination of the peritoneum that normally obliterates during development.

A. This describes direct inguinal hernias. Hesselbach's triangle consists of the lateral border of the rectus abdominus muscle, the inguinal ligament, and the inferior epigastric vessels.
B. Indirect inguinal hernias always pass through the deep inguinal ring.
D. Weakening of the conjoint tendon contributes to the development of direct inguinal hernias.
E. Indirect inguinal hernias are the most common hernia in both males and females.

155. B This is a presentation of schizophrenia. Schizophrenia is commonly associated with a prodrome phase with a decline in daily tasks and withdrawal from social activities and then, later, positive (hallucinations, delusions) and negative (apathy, withdrawal, flattening of affect) symptoms. The newer atypical antipsychotic medications are thusly named because they do not have similar chemical structures, while the typical antipsychotics do bear chemical and structural similarities.

A. The opposite is true: the positive symptoms respond better to the typical antipsychotics than the negative symptoms.

C. Most commonly schizophrenia will follow a progressively deteriorating course. Although it has been found that proper social support can slow this rate of decline, most patients will never regain their pre-illness level of functioning.

D. Long-term family and social support is a necessary part of the psychosocial treatment in schizophrenia in order to maximize quality of life and level of functioning in society.

E. Parkinsonian-type (extra-pyramidal) symptoms are associated with the typical antipsychotics.

156. A Steroids act by diffusing through the cell membrane and binding to specific cytoplasmic transcription factors. These transcription factors then move to the nucleus to enhance transcription of specific genes. It takes several hours for the production of target proteins to be influenced by the administration of steroid hormones.

B. This describes the mechanism of many non-steroidal hormones, which act more rapidly by acting on cell surface receptors to initiate signalization cascades.

C. Steroids work through transcription factors, not directly.

D. Differential processing of mRNA is not a part of steroid action.

157. A The physician should suspect *Neisseria meningitidis*, which is a gram-negative diplococcus. This bacterium is prevalent in crowded places like college dormitories. It will cause symptoms of headache, fever, and coma. Cerebrospinal fluid will usually have increased PMNs, low glucose, and increased protein.

B. This describes either an enterococcus or group D-nonenterococcus. These are responsible for urinary tract infections and subacute bacterial endocarditis.

C. This is a description of *Staphylococcus saprophyticus*. This is responsible for urinary tract infections.

D. Western equine encephalitis is from the Togaviridae family and is responsible for a viral encephalitis, not a bacterial one. It would result in an increase in lymphocytes, increased protein content, unaltered glucose levels, and unaltered CSF pressure.

E. Measles virus also causes viral encephalitis and leads to a special condition called subacute sclerosing panencephalitis.

158. E Chloramphenicol works on the 50s ribosomal subunit. Its action would most likely be unaffected by a change in a bacteria's 30s ribosomal subunit.

A, B, C, and **D** are incorrect. All of these antibiotics work on the 30s ribosomal subunit.

159. D The patient most likely has Horner's syndrome (ptosis, anhidrosis, and miosis) due to an apical bronchogenic carcinoma. Symptoms such as ptosis (drooping of the eyelid), miosis (narrowing of the pupil of the eye), anhidrosis, enophthalmos, and loss of ciliospinal reflex are caused by interruption of the sympathetic nerve fibers of the cervical sympathetic ganglia by either the mass effect or malignancy of the carcinoma.

A. The levator palpebrae superioris muscle elevates the upper eyelid and is innervated by CN III (oculomotor nerve) and sympathetic nerve. The clinical presentation does not suggest CN III damage.

B. CN IV (trochlear) innervates the superior oblique muscle.

C. CN VI (abducens) innervates the lateral rectus muscle. Mnemonics SO_4LR_6

E. CN II (optic) is a sensory neuron dealing with vision.

160. A Tetralogy of Fallot is characterized by pulmonary stenosis (obstruction of the right ventricular outflow tract), ventricular septal defect, dextroposition of the aorta (overriding the septum), and right ventricular hypertrophy. Patients become cyanotic due to the right to left shunting across the VSD and decrease in pulmonary flow.

B. Is incorrect. See A.

C. Is incorrect. See A, also the EKG shows right axis deviation, which is consistent with right ventricular hypertrophy, not left.

D. Is incorrect. See A and C.

E. Is incorrect. See A.

161. C Patients with histrionic personality disorder have a need to be the center of attention. They often dress dramatically and inappropriately, are excessively emotional, and display inappropriately seductive behavior.

A. Patients with antisocial personality disorder show disregard for social norms. They often break the law, act in an aggressive manner, are deceitful, and have no remorse for their actions.

B. Patients with schizoid personality disorder prefer to be alone and derive little pleasure from social contacts. They have difficulty expressing emotions and do not generally seek relationships.

D. Although patients with avoidant personality disorder desire relationships, they usually avoid them because they experience anxiety and a fear of rejection due to feelings of inadequacy. As a result, they are often socially isolated.

E. Although patients with dependent personality disorder are abnormally dependent on others, these patients are generally passive, isolated people who are sensitive to criticism and have difficulty making decisions.

162. D Carbon monoxide is bad for two reasons. First, it binds to hemoglobin 200 to 250 times more than oxygen. Second, it causes whatever oxygen is bound to hemoglobin to stay bound to hemoglobin, creating a left shift in the oxygen-hemoglobin dissociation curve. Note that blood with 60% of its hemoglobin as HbCO and 40% of its hemoglobin as HbO_2 has a greater affinity for oxygen than does blood with only 40% of HbO_2 and 0% HbCO (as is the case found in anemia). The anemia curve is shifted to the right while the COHb curves are altered in shape, more closely resembling a hyperbola than a sigmoid. Thus, carbon monoxide not only decreases the total oxygen carrying capacity of blood by rendering a portion of the hemoglobin binding sites unusable to oxygen, but also it shifts the oxygen-hemoglobin dissociation curve of the remaining hemoglobin to the left by binding oxygen more avidly. This further starves the tissues and organs of vital oxygen supplies. Therefore, the curve with the greatest percentage of carbon monoxide will bind oxygen with the greatest affinity.

A, B, C, and E are incorrect. See explanation above.

163 E *Pseudomonas aeruginosa* is a common organism responsible for soft tissue infections in diabetics. It classically produces a blue-green tinted pus and an odor described as either like "grape juice" or "taco shells." It is also a common cause of "swimmer's ear" (otitis externa).

A. Although *Staph aureus* is a common skin pathogen, it produces a golden pus and a foul-smelling odor if any odor is present. It is also a gram-positive cocci.

B. *Proteus vulgaris* is rarely a soft tissue pathogen.

C. *C. perfringens* usually produces a foul odor with a dark brown pus. It is also gram positive.

D. *Strep pyogenes* is gram positive.

164. E Lisinopril is an ACE inhibitor. An ACE inhibitor when used with an NSAID may cause too great of a vasodilatory effect on the kidney, potentially leading to kidney failure.

A. Furosemide does not have a large potential interaction with chronic NSAID use.

B. Nifedipine has no contraindications with NSAID use.

C. Methyldopa has no contraindications with NSAID use.

D. Clonidine has no contraindications with NSAID use.

165. A Huntington's disease, an autosomal dominant, chromosome 4, progressive disease, usually begins in young to middle age and is characterized by choreiform movements and dementia. Neuroanatomic findings are bilateral wasting of the putamen and head of the caudate nucleus, which correlate to the neurochemical loss of GABA-ergic neurons.

B. Schizophrenia is associated with increased dopaminergic activity.

C. Parkinson's disease is associated with decreased dopaminergic activity.

D. Alzheimer's disease is associated with decreased acetylcholine activity.

E. Depression is associated with decreased serotonin levels.

166. E The patient had tertiary syphilis, whose pathognomonic features include Argyll-Robertson pupils (pupils that do not react to light, but only to near-accommodation). The causative organism is *Treponema pallidum*.

A. *Mycobacterium tuberculosis* is the cause of tuberculosis.
B. *B. burgdorferi* is the cause of Lyme disease. Acutely, Lyme disease causes fever, chills, fatigue, headache, muscle and joint pain, lymphadenopathy, and a characteristic rash. Long-term sequelae include arthritis, cardiac dysrhythmias, and nervous system abnormalities.
C. *Legionella pneumophila* is the cause of Legionnaire's disease, a pneumonia.
D. *Francisella tularensis* is the cause of tularemia. Tularemia presents with fever, headache, and an ulcerated skin lesion with localized lymph node enlargement. It may also present with eye infection, GI ulcerations, or pneumonia.

167. B With vomiting, the pH becomes elevated due to loss of H^+ from the stomach, resulting in metabolic alkalosis. Since Cl^- is lost along with the H^+, hypochloremia occurs. Loss of HCl results in ECF volume contraction, decreased blood volume, decreased renal perfusion pressure, and increased renin secretion, resulting in increased aldosterone levels. Increased aldosterone results in increased K^+ secretion by the distal tubules, leading to hypokalemia. The metabolic alkalosis due to vomiting has resulted in respiratory compensation by the patient (low respiratory rate and therefore increased pCO_2).

A. Respiratory alkalosis is caused by a primary increase in respiratory rate and a loss of CO_2. In this case, the primary cause of alkalosis was metabolic (vomiting), and compensation resulted in a decreased respiratory rate, not increased.
C. Respiratory acidosis is characterized by a low pH and is caused by a primary decrease in respiratory rate resulting in retention of CO_2. In this case, the pH is elevated and the decrease in respiratory rate was secondary, not primary, to compensate for the metabolic alkalosis.
D. Metabolic acidosis is characterized by a low pH and can be due to several causes: ketoacidosis, chronic renal failure, and diarrhea, as well as others. The respiratory compensation for metabolic

acidosis is hyperventilation. In this case, the pH is elevated and the respiratory compensation was hypoventilation.
E. The pH, pCO_2, and $[HCO_3^-]$ values are all abnormal, so this person cannot have a normal acid-base status.

168. D Flumazenil, a benzodiazepine analog, competitively inhibits the actions of benzodiazepines at benzodiazepine receptors in the central nervous system, therefore reversing the CNS effects of benzodiazepines.

A. Naloxone is an antidote for opioid analgesics.
B. Edetate is an antidote for lead.
C. Deferoxamine is an antidote for iron salts.
E. Acetylcysteine is an antidote for acetaminophen.

169. D Human Papillomavirus 16 (HPV-16) is associated with cervical carcinoma. Human Papillomavirus 18 (HPV-18) is also associated with cervical carcinoma.

A. Human Papillomavirus 1 (HPV-1) is the causative agent of the plantar wart and is not associated with human malignancy.
B. Human Papillomavirus 6 (HPV-6) is a common cause of condyloma acuminatum (genital warts) and is not associated with human malignancy.
C. Human Papillomavirus 11 (HPV-11), together with HPV-6, accounts for approximately 90% of genital warts. Neither is associated with human malignancy.
E. Epstein-Barr virus (EBV) is associated with nasopharyngeal carcinoma and with African Burkitt's lymphoma.

170. D Vitamin C (ascorbic acid) is present in fresh fruits and vegetables and is necessary for the hydroxylation of proline to hydroxyproline in collagen. This process is necessary for the maintenance of connective tissue containing collagen.

A. Insulin production is not affected by vitamin C deficiency.
B. These coagulation factors are dependent on the presence of vitamin K.
C. Globin production is not dependent on vitamin C.

171. E Panic attacks are characterized by intense periods of anxiety or fear that start suddenly and generally last up to 30 minutes. Symptoms may include sweating, chest pain, palpitations, nausea, choking sensation, trembling, and fears of losing control or dying. By definition the attack must last 10 minutes or more.

A. Specific phobias are excessive or unreasonable fears brought on by the presence of a specific object or being. The individual is able to recognize that the fear is excessive.

B. Viral illness is very unlikely given the brief and episodic nature of this presentation.

C. Malingering is the conscious feigning of a disorder in order to obtain a specific gain. Gain in this case could be getting out of exams or attaining different exam conditions, although this is unlikely given her intent to get treatment and continue toward her goal.

D. Formaldehyde allergy would not present in this manner; additionally the woman experienced the symptoms in a completely different context during the physiology exam.

172. E This patient most probably has a lactic acidosis. The ABG shows a metabolic acidosis with mild respiratory compensation. The patient's increased respiratory rate confirms that there is a respiratory compensation. The electrolytes show an elevated anion gap that occurs with lactic acidosis. There is also an elevated creatinine, suggesting some degree of renal insufficiency. Of the drugs listed, only metformin is known to cause lactic acidosis, especially in patients with renal insufficiency.

A. Glyburide is a sulfonylurea, and its most common side effect is hypoglycemia.

B. Rosiglitazone is a newer antidiabetic agent that increases peripheral insulin sensitivity. Common adverse reactions are hepatotoxicity and CHF exacerbation.

C. Insulin is not a first-line agent in type II diabetics and is not known to cause lactic acidosis. Its most common side effect is hypoglycemia.

D. Acarbose prevents carbohydrate absorption in the intestine and can cause flatulence and diarrhea.

173. C Thiazide diuretics, such as hydrochlorothiazide and chlorothiazide, inhibit NaCl reabsorption in the early distal tubule, decreasing the diluting capacity of the nephron. Common reactions include dizziness, headache, fatigue, and musculoskeletal pain. Signs of toxicity include hypokalemia, metabolic alkalosis, hyponatremia, hyperglycemia, hyperlipidemia, hyperuricemia, and hypercalcemia.

A. Spironolactone, a K^+-sparing diuretic, is a competitive aldosterone receptor antagonist. Side effects include hyperkalemia and gynecomastia.

B. Furosemide is a loop-diuretic that inhibits the cotransport system (Na, K, $2Cl^-$) of the thick ascending limb of the loop of Henle. Side effects include hypokalemia, hyperuricemia, and hypocalcemia.

D. Triamterene is also a K^+-sparing diuretic and acts by blocking Na^+ channels in the collecting tubule. Side effects include hyperkalemia.

E. Mechanism of action is similar to that of furosemide. Side effects include hypokalemia and hypocalcemia but not hyperuricemia.

174. D Motor innervation of vastus medialis is via the femoral nerve; all other listed muscles are innervated by the sciatic nerve. Given the lesion's location it would be likely all the other muscles would be affected to some degree. Biceps femoris would be affected by wallerian degeneration, as the proximal axon to the damage undergoes degeneration secondary to the primary lesion.

A. Gastrocnemius is innervated by the sciatic nerve.

B. Biceps femoris is innervated by the sciatic nerve.

C. Tibialis anterior is innervated by the sciatic nerve.

175. C Low concentration of the serotonin metabolite 5-hydroxy-indoleacetic acid (5-HIAA) has been linked to suicidal behavior in several studies.

A. Increased protein has not been shown to be linked with increased suicide.

B. The presence of RBCs has not been shown to be linked with increased suicide.

D. Increased 5-HIAA has not been shown to be linked with increased suicide.

E. Decreased glucose has not been shown to be linked with increased suicide.

176. C The generation time of a bacterium is the same as its doubling time. In each generation time, the bacterium undergoes binary fission in which one bacterium becomes two. So, in three generation times the flask will become filled (assuming that optimum growth requirements have been met). This question is getting at the basic notion that exponential growth can become "out of hand" quite rapidly.

A. In 20 minutes the flask will be one-fourth filled.
B. In 40 minutes the flask will be one-half filled.
D. In 2 hours there would be enough bacteria to fill 8 flasks.
E. In 4 hours there would be enough bacteria to fill 512 flasks.

177. E Older patients often are taking multiple daily medications. The clinician must be aware of possible interactions. The elderly lose body size, so if the same amount of drug is administered, the body concentration may be higher. The elderly lose body water and gain body fat, which again affects the drug concentration and distribution. As most functions decrease with age, so do phase 1 reactions. Finally, cysts appear in the kidneys and nephrons one by one stop functioning and renal blood flow decreases. This may increase drug concentration due to reduced elimination by the kidneys.

A, B, C, D are incorrect. See E above.

178. D Goodpasture's syndrome usually occurs in young men. Hemoptysis and hematuria are due to inflammation in the basement membranes of the lungs and the kidney due to autoantibodies to the basement membranes. The course of the disease is rapid. Treatment includes reduction of inflammation and removal of the antibodies.

A. This pattern is seen in acute post-streptococcal glomerulonephritis and membranous glomerulonephritis.
B. This pattern is seen in rapidly progressive (crescentic) glomerulonephritis.
C. This pattern is seen in IgA nephropathy (Berger's disease).

179. D Fluoroquinolone antibiotics act by inhibition of DNA gyrase, an enzyme necessary for unwinding of double-stranded DNA in bacteria. Resistance occurs when genes encoding DNA gyrase are altered or the bacteria are able to remove the antibiotic from their intracellular space.

A. Production of β-lactamase is a mechanism of resistance to penicillin and related antibiotics that act at the bacterial cell wall.
B. The 50S ribosomal subunit is the target of other antibiotics, including the macrolides and clindamycin.
C. The 30S ribosomal subunit is the target of other antibiotics, including the aminoglycosides and tetracycline.

180. B Open-ended questions are the most likely to establish rapport and a good relationship with patients, although are often more time consuming. Less structure is given to the patient and they are more likely to speak freely, which often discloses important information in other areas. Obviously there are certain specialties in which open-ended questions are more useful, such as in psychiatry as compared with surgery.

A, B, C, and E are all direct questions.

181. D According to the Poiseuille-Hagen formula, resistance of a cylinder varies inversely with the fourth power of the radius ($r4$). Flow varies inversely with the resistance of the vessel. Since resistance is increased 16-fold, blood flow will be reduced to 1/16 of original flow.

A, B, C, and E are incorrect, since $1/2^4 = 1/16$.

182. C Thiazide diuretics are very effective in nephrogenic diabetes insipidus. Their mechanism of action is to inhibit the reabsorption of sodium and chloride in the early distal renal tubule.

A. Lypressin is administered intranasally, has a duration of four to six hours, and is used in pituitary deficiency diabetes insipidus.
B. Vasopressin can be given IM, and can cause HTN. It is used in pituitary deficiency diabetes insipidus.
D. Desmopressin (DDAVP) is administered intranasally and lasts about 12 hours without increasing the blood pressure. It is used in pituitary deficiency diabetes insipidus.

183. C This patient has a case of vaginitis caused by *Gardnerella*. The foul-smelling discharge and clue cells on smear (epithelial cells with dots) are classically found in *Gardnerella* vaginitis. The latter are pathognomonic for this organism.

A. Although *Candida* is the most common cause of vaginitis, there is usually a cheesy-white discharge and pseudohyphae would be seen under the microscope. There would not be any clue cells.

B. *Trichomonas* is another common cause of vaginitis, but it also would not present with clue cells. It also causes a green, frothy discharge and severe pruritus.

D. *Neisseria* can present with urethritis, cervicitis, or PID. However, clue cells are not found.

E. *Chlamydia* can cause the same symptoms as *Neisseria*, but again there would be no clue cells.

184. C The formation of a femoral vein hematoma is a serious complication. Typically, patients will have pain at the site and an expanding mass with decreased peripheral pulses. The important anatomy in this region is that the vein, artery, and nerve travel parallel in that order from medial to lateral. The peripheral pulse may well decrease due to compression of the femoral artery.

A. The hematocrit will either stay the same or decrease secondary to an acute bleed (although this may not be detected for six or more hours).

B. The blood pressure may drop secondary to decreased blood volume.

D. The temperature may drop secondary to decreased blood flow and vasoconstriction of the vascular bed.

185. B Intoxication with cocaine is characterized by euphoria, agitation, hallucinations, and impaired judgment. On physical exam, a patient will often present with dilated pupils, hypertension, and tachycardia. One hour after using cocaine, the patient will become lethargic and the euphoria will be gone.

A. Heroin withdrawal is characterized by flulike symptoms: sweating, piloerection, fever, rhinorrhea, nausea, abdominal pains, and diarrhea. Patients also present with anxiety, insomnia, yawning, and pupillary dilation.

C. Amphetamine withdrawal is characterized by lethargy, dysphoria, depression, and fatigue.

D. Phencyclidine (PCP) intoxication, also known as "angel dust," is characterized by violent behavior, vertical or horizontal nystagmus, fever, agitation, psychosis, and delirium.

E. Lysergic acid diethylamide (LSD) intoxication is characterized by anxiety or depression, delusions, visual hallucinations, flashbacks, diaphoresis, and palpitations.

186. B HMG-CoA reductase inhibitors such as lovastatin ("statins") slow the rate-limiting step in hepatic cholesterol biosynthesis. This action indirectly leads to an increase in LDL receptor levels and enhanced clearance of LDL cholesterol from the circulation.

A. This describes the action of the bile acid binding resins colestipol and cholestyramine, other cholesterol-lowering drugs.

C. This describes the action of orlistat, a drug used to treat obesity.

D. This describes the mechanism of fibric acid derivatives, other cholesterol-lowering drugs.

187. A This patient's symptoms are consistent with orthostatic (or postural) hypotension. In this patient with no obvious blood loss or dehydration, autonomic insufficiency is the most likely reason for orthostatic hypotension. Elderly, diabetic patients are at greatly increased risk of autonomic insufficiency, which can be confirmed by measuring blood pressure in the supine, seated, and standing positions.

B. Sensory neuropathy may lead to decreased balance, but would not be expected to cause lightheadedness and fainting.

C. Cerebrovascular accidents, or strokes, produce neurologic signs and symptoms that persist following the event.

D. Peripheral vascular disease does not cause lightheadedness or fainting.

188. E This patient has acquired autoimmune deficiency syndrome (AIDS) and is currently being treated with triple antiretroviral therapy against HIV. The new guidelines for the latest antiretroviral treatment recommendations can be found at www.hivatis.org. In this case, the history of IV drug abuse, the picture of Kaposi's sarcoma, and the long treatment history of five months highly suggests HIV infection. The patient is likely following a highly active antiretroviral therapy (HAART) plan that includes combinations of one or more of a nucleoside reverse transcriptase inhibitor (NRTI), a nonnucleoside reverse transcriptase inhibitor (NNRTI), and protease inhibitor (PI). The patient presents to the ED with an acute kidney stone (nephrolithiasis) attack and a subsequent finding of protease inhibitor associated lipodystrophy (PIAL). Indinavir is a protease inhibitor specifically associated with nephrolithiasis, especially when patients do not receive adequate hydration.

A. ZDV (previously known as AZT) is a NRTI that has a short-term side effect of bone marrow suppression with anemia.

B. ddC is an NRTI that causes peripheral neuropathy, aphthous oral ulcers (stomatitis), and maculovesicular cutaneous eruptions.

C. Abacavir is an NRTI which is a guanine analog that causes hypersensitivity reactions with flulike symptoms and skin rashes.

D. Efavirenz is an NNRTI with the most common complication of skin rashes and increased liver enzymes.

189. E Urinary incontinence, gait ataxia, and forgetfulness are clues that should lead one to suspect normal-pressure hydrocephalus. A CT of the head should be ordered for confirmation.

A. Elderly patients with hypothyroidism may show symptoms of dementia and weight gain.

B. Head trauma may have several different manifestations of symptoms depending on the mechanism of injury and the anatomical structures affected.

C. Small handwriting is one of the manifestations of Parkinson's disease, not normal-pressure hydrocephalus.

D. Forgetfulness is one of the symptoms of dementia. It does not give any specific clues as to the cause of the dementia.

F. Head trauma may lead to urinary urgency, but it would be unrelated to the above condition.

190. B Although the ELISA test is very sensitive, it does give false positive results at times. To decrease this chance, a second ELISA test is done. If this is positive, confirmation is still needed in the form of the Western blot test. This test looks for antibodies in the patient's serum to the HIV antigens *gag*, *pol*, and *env*. A positive Western blot test confirms the diagnosis of HIV infection.

A. Since two ELISA tests have been done and have both been positive, there is no need to do another one. It adds nothing to the first two, and a Western blot test would still be needed.

C. This is the treatment for HIV, but should not be started before the diagnosis is confirmed with the Western blot test.

D. Again, treatment of any sort should not begin before confirming the ELISA test results. Furthermore, Bactrim prophylaxis for PCP is usually not begun until the CD4 count is below 200.

E. HIV patients do not need any special type of contact precautions beyond standard precautions to prevent transmission of blood-borne pathogens.

191. A This infant has the most common form of congenital adrenal hyperplasia, 21-alpha-hydroxylase deficiency. In this disorder of steroid biosynthesis, the patient is unable to synthesize aldosterone or cortisol; intermediates are, instead, shunted back, resulting in the synthesis of androstenedione and testosterone. In a genetic 46 XX female, these elevated androgen levels result in virilization of the external genitalia, converting the labia into a penis-like organ, even though internally the patient remains a female. Salt wasting and hypotension due to mineralcorticoid deficiency typically present by the second week of life.

B. While 11-beta-hydroxylase deficiency does result in virilization from the same shunting mechanism as 21-alpha-hydroxylase deficiency, these patients are able to synthesize 11-deoxycorticosterone. Thus, unlike 21-alpha-hydroxylase deficiency patients, 11-beta-hydroxylase deficiency patients are hypertensive and salt-retaining.

C. 17-alpha-hydroxylase deficiency patients who are 46 XX are not virilized because androstenedione and testosterone cannot be synthesized.

D. Homogentisic oxidase deficiency results in alcaptonuria.

E. Alpha-L-iduronidase deficiency results in Hurler's syndrome, characterized by heparin sulfate and dematan sulfate accumulation in the viscera.

192. C This question is open-ended and general. The patient can speak freely about her headache or anywhere else that is hurting.

A. This is a closed-ended question and gives the patient a limited choice of responses.

B. Again this is a closed-ended question and gives the patient a limited choice of responses.

D. This start ignores the patient's primary complaint at the outset of the encounter.

E. This question is too narrow and focused for the start of the clinical interview.

193. A Phenytoin is used to suppress tonic-clinic and partial seizures. It can cause gingival hyperplasia and coarsening of facial features, especially in children.

B. Carbamazepine is also used to suppress tonic-clonic and partial seizures. It can cause severe side effects such as aplastic anemia, agranulocytosis, thrombocytopenia, and liver toxicity.

C. Phenobarbital is used in simple partial seizures and tonic-clonic seizures. Adverse effects are rash, nausea, vomiting, and sedation.

D. Valproic acid is used in myoclonic seizures and general tonic-clonic seizures. It can cause hepatic toxicity and rash.

E. Clonazepam is a benzodiazapine that is effective in myoclonic and absence seizures. It has sedative side effects.

194. E Symptoms described are classic for vitamin C deficiency, also known as scurvy.

A. Vitamin A deficiency leads to dry skin and night blindness.

B. Vitamin B_1 deficiency (thiamine deficiency) is common in alcoholics and leads to beriberi and Wernicke-Korsakoff syndrome.

C. Deficiency in vitamin B_2 leads to angular stomatitis and cheilosis.

D. Deficiency in vitamin B_6 is seen in patients taking INH. Symptoms are convulsions and irritability.

F. Vitamin D is related to [Ca++] regulation. Deficiency in children leads to rickets. Deficiency in adults leads to osteomalacia.

G. Vitamin E deficiency leads to anemia secondary to increased fragility of erythrocytes.

195. C The scratch from two days ago with mild wound infection but profound descending weakness and paralysis is associated with *Clostridium botulinum* wound infection. Here, spores contaminate a wound, germinate, and produce toxin at the site of infection. While this is a feasible route, it is most common in the United States to get wound botulism via drug abuse, especially skin-popping with black tar heroin. The second route of spread is mostly found in infants and is associated with ingestion of preformed toxin within foods (honey most commonly cited). The treatment is trivalent antitoxin (A, B, and E) and respiratory support. Antitoxin is made in horses and is associated with a 15% serum sickness reaction rate.

A. Without therapy this illness will result in complete paralysis, including respiratory muscles, and death will follow. Supportive treatment could be appropriate for specific cases of Guillain-Barré syndrome, which is the most common cause of paralysis in the United States. However, that would follow an infectious illness and the paralysis is described as rapidly progressive ascending. Treatment of moderate to severe Guillian-Barré is IVIG or plasmaphoresis as needed.

B. Vaccination is used for prevention of many illnesses, but is not a method of treatment (nor even prevention in this case). Prevention of infection is by proper sterilization of canned foods.

D. Debridement is treatment of choice for the *Clostridium perfringens* infection and associated gas gangrene. In that case, pain, edema, and crepitus at the site of the wound would be the most likely symptoms, and descending paralysis is not seen as a common presentation.

E. Antibiotics are not helpful in treatment of the above infection.

196. D Sickle cell anemia occurs as a result of a mutation in the beta-globin gene of the hemoglobin molecule. In sickle cell trait (i.e., the carrier state), only one mutant allele for this gene is inherited, while the other inherited allele is normal. In sickle cell disease, both inherited alleles are mutated. It is common to test for this disease via amniocentesis using the dot blot technique. In this technique the patient's DNA is amplified by PCR and spotted onto two areas of a filter. An ASO probe designed to anneal with the mutant form of the gene is applied to one area, and a probe designed to anneal with the normal gene is applied to the other. The dot blot is then photographed and visualized (using fluorescent antibodies attached to the probes). If the blot of DNA with the normal probe lights up (turning the blot black on film), and the other doesn't, then neither of the patient's alleles contains a mutation. If the blot of DNA with the probe to the mutant allele lights up, and the other doesn't, then both of the patient's alleles are mutated. If both blots light up, you know the patient is a carrier, having one normal allele and one mutant allele. In this clinical scenario we are told that the father has the disease, but are not told the exact genetic status of the mother. Although we can safely assume she has never had the disease (given that she has never manifested any of its symptoms), we cannot rule out the possibility that she may be a carrier. This answer represents one of the possible results that could have been obtained from this family. It shows a father who has sickle cell disease (as the clinical scenario indicates), a mother who is a carrier (which the data given allow for), and a fetus who is a carrier. It is certainly possible for these parents to produce such a fetus, and is in fact the best you could hope for, given their genetic makeup.

A and **B.** If the mother were to have two normal alleles and the father two mutant ones, every child they would ever have would turn out to be a carrier. Such a fetus could never be completely normal nor have sickle cell disease. Answer A is impossible because it shows a fetus with parents of this genetic makeup having two normal alleles. Answer B is impossible because it shows a fetus with the same such parents, having two mutant alleles.

C. If the mother were to have one normal and one mutant allele (with a father having two abnormal alleles), 50% of the children would become carriers and 50% would inherit two mutant alleles and have the disease. But, a fetus of parents with such a genetic makeup could never be normal. Since this answer shows a normal fetus with parents of this genetic makeup, it is impossible.

E. This dot blot indicates that the father has one normal and one mutant allele, although the clinical scenario clearly indicates that the father has sickle cell disease, which by definition implies two mutant alleles.

197. E Bioavailability is the fraction of administered drug that reaches systemic circulation. This is affected by numerous factors including changes that occur to the drug when in the body, and the nature of the drugs chemical composition and stability.

A. Many drugs undergo significant change during passage through the liver.

B. Drugs that are extremely hydrophobic have difficulty becoming soluble in cells, and drugs that are extremely hydrophilic have difficulty crossing cell membranes.

C. How well a drug dissolves is affected by how it is formulated.

D. Some drugs are broken down during their passage through the body because of their unstable properties.

198. D The description found here is classic for disseminated coccidioidomycosis. The organism responsible for this disease state is *Coccidioides immitis*, a thermally dimorphic fungus growing as a mold at 25 degrees C and as spherules full of endospores in host tissue (37° C). The mold, which is inhaled from the environment, exists in the form of thick-walled, barrel-shaped spores (arthrospores). This fungus is endemic to the southwestern United States and northern portions of Mexico, extending from Texas to California. The primary infection is usually asymptomatic, though some develop mild to severe upper respiratory infections or lobar pneumonia (as seen in the right upper lung field in this patient). Others can develop a chronic, progressive pulmonary coccidioidomycosis. A small pleural effusion might also be present, as well as hilar lymphadenopathy. Some patients can develop hypersensitivity reactions, one of which presents as erythema nodosum, which the above patient demonstrates on his lower extremities. Dissemination is more likely to occur in African-Americans, Filipinos, Native Americans, Mexican-Americans, pregnant women (especially third trimester) and the immunosuppressed. It can disseminate to bone, skin, meninges (as in our patient), subcutaneous tissue, and joints, as well as other sites. CSF examination usually does not reveal the organism, though CSF findings are classic for fungal meningitis.

A. This applies to *Histoplasma capsulatum*, the agent responsible for histoplasmosis.

B. This also applies to *Histoplasma capsulatum* and not *Coccidioides immitis*.

C. This is necessary to diagnose *Pneumocystis carinii* infection, not coccidioidomycosis.

E. AIDS patients with CD4+ counts less than 200/uL are at increased risk for infections with *Pneumocystis carinii*, so much so that they need to receive prophylactic antibiotic treatment (trimethoprim/sulfamethoxazole) when their CD4+ counts are this low. Prophylactic treatment against *Coccidioides immitis* is not indicated.

199. D Turner's syndrome is the result of losing one sex chromosome during development. The incidence is about 1 in 4000 live female births. This 15-year-old girl displays the classic picture of Turner's syndrome: short stature, webbed neck, wide and broad chest, amenorrhea, failure of development of secondary sex characteristics, and short fourth metacarpal. In addition to these physical findings, additional manifestations can include: ptosis, hypoplasia of the nails, aortic coarctation, bicuspid aortic valve, and renal or gastrointestinal disorders.

A. A 46, XX genotype results in a normal female.

B. A 47, XXY genotype results in a male with Klinefelter's syndrome. These tall patients exhibit symptoms on a broad continuum from serious learning disabilities to above average intellect. Other physical findings include gynecomastia, long arms and legs, and sparse facial hair.

C. A 47, XYY genotype results in a male with an increased propensity for behavioral, learning, and attention disorders. These patients usually have no physical abnormalities.

E. A 47, XXX genotype results in a female with an increased likelihood of sterility and menstrual irregularities.

200. A Endotoxemia and activation of the complement system are correct. Septic shock described in this question is commonly seen with gram-negative septicemia. Endotoxin released from the cell walls of certain gram-negative bacteria, such as *E. coli* (most common cause of gram-negative sepsis) produces the findings described in this question.

B. Endotoxins stimulate mononuclear blood cells to increase tumor necrosis factor-alpha and IL-1 release, thus producing damage to endothelial cells.

C. Anaphylotoxins get activated, vasodilating peripheral blood vessels, and thus producing warm but dry skin. In addition, increased vasodilation increases venous return with increase in cardiac output. Hence, a common cause of high-output failure.

D and **E** are incorrect as they describe processes opposite of that occurring in septic shock.

So, to review common types of shock,

Hypovolemic shock is associated with low cardiac output and high systemic resistance.

Cardiogenic is associated with high pulmonary capillary wedge pressure.

Neurogenic is associated with low systemic vascular resistance, venous oxygen saturation, wedge pressure, and systemic vascular resistance.

Septic is the only type of shock associated with high cardiac output and high systemic venous O_2 but low resistance and capillary wedge pressure.

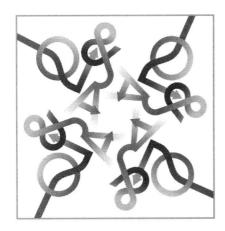

QUESTIONS
BLOCK 5

201. You are a medical student completing an overnight rotation in the respiratory care unit. Five new patients are admitted, and the attending physician hands you the following arterial blood gas measurements. With a sense of urgency, the physician requests that you immediately place oxygen therapy on one of the patients. Which patient is the most hypoxemic?

	Hb (g/dL)	SaO_2 (%)	PaO_2 (mm Hg)
A. Patient A	7	95	85
B. Patient B	15	85	55
C. Patient C	15	70	85
D. Patient D	14	85	82
E. Patient E	6	98	100

202. A 45-year-old horse farm worker is brought to the emergency room one summer day with a five-day history of increasing muscle spasms. On the day of admission he is virtually rigid due to the spasms. History and physical do not reveal any accident or definite wound site. What is the likely cause of this man's muscle spasms?

A. *Clostridium perfringens*
B. *Clostridium tetani*
C. *Clostridium botulinum*
D. *Clostridium difficile*
E. None of the above

203. A 54-year-old black male presents to your office with a history of smoking two packs of cigarettes per day for the past 30 years. He has a productive cough most of the time, which has been present for at least three years. Sputum culture failed to grow any pathogenic organisms. Chest x-ray does not reveal any mass lesions. He is afebrile, and a CBC was within normal limits. What treatment regimen would you prescribe?

A. Salmeterol, corticosteroids, and theophylline
B. Cromolyn sodium, corticosteroids, and theophylline
C. Albuterol, theophylline, and corticosteroids
D. Ipratropium bromide, albuterol, and theophylline
E. Albuterol, zileuton, and corticosteroids

204. An 81-year-old female fell and fractured her hip. She has been hospitalized for two weeks since the accident. Over the past few days she has become increasingly confused and forgetful. She has torn out her IV in an attempt to "get the snakes out of her bed," and is distrustful and fights with the staff, stating she thinks they are trying to poison her with the wrong medications. Before her hospitalization she was living with her husband in a retirement community and has been generally in good health. The most likely diagnosis is:

A. Alzheimer's disease
B. Parkinson's disease
C. Schizophrenia
D. Delirium
E. Delirium tremens

205. A 46-year-old female presents to her primary care provider with a history of painful, dry eyes and dry mouth that have been getting worse for the last three years. She also has a history of Hashimoto's thyroiditis. Blood tests reveal the presence of RF antibodies, ANA antibodies, and anti SS-A and SS-B antibodies. The most likely disease affecting this patient is:

A. SLE
B. Rheumatoid arthritis
C. Systemic sclerosis
D. Sjögren's syndrome
E. CREST syndrome

206. A 40-year-old female of Native American descent is scheduled for an elective cholecystectomy. Your attending begins to ask you questions about the anatomy of the biliary system. **(See Figure 206.)** Which of the following is true?

   A. The arterial supply of the gallbladder usually arises from the right hepatic artery.

   B. The cystic duct empties directly into the duodenum.

   C. Bile is produced and stored in the gallbladder.

   D. The gallbladder is a retroperitoneal organ.

   E. The sphincter of Oddi is located in the common bile duct and prevents retrograde flow of bile into the right and left hepatic ducts.

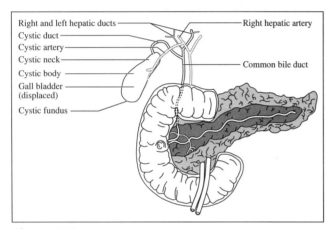

Figure 206

207. A 45-year-old Caucasian male appears in your office complaining of pain and swelling in his left knee. He says that this has happened before, in his knees and in other joints of his legs and feet, all episodes eventually resolving in a few days. This is the worst it has ever been. Upon examination, he has a temperature of 101.1 degrees and a reddened, swollen, warm left knee joint, very tender to touch. Gram's stain and culture of the synovial fluid are negative. Synovial fluid WBC count is 50,000/mm³ (normal <200/mm³). Examination of the synovial fluid under red-compensated, polarized light reveals needle-shaped negatively birefringent crystals. Some are seen present within neutrophils. A uric acid blood level comes back 5 mg/dL (normal 3.5–7.2 mg/dL).

Which of the following statements is true concerning the biochemical pathway responsible for producing the metabolite that is accumulating in this patient's knee?

   A. Hereditary fructose intolerance has been associated with increased activity of the pathway in question, and subsequent manifestation of the above disease.

   B. The product formed by the enzyme deficient in severe combined immunodeficiency (SCID) is hypoxanthine.

   C. Increased conversion of 5-phosphoribosylamine to inosine monophosphate (IMP) results in an increase in the synthesis and subsequent degradation of AMP and GMP, often leading to the disease state seen above.

   D. During the conversion of 5-phosphoribosylamine to IMP, only a portion of the amino acid glycine is incorporated into the IMP purine ring.

   E. The purine ring undergoes considerable formation and refinement before being placed upon the activated form of ribose-5-phosphate during de novo purine synthesis, unlike in pyrimidine synthesis where the activated ribose-5-phosphate molecule serves as an early foundation upon which the purine ring is built.

208. A 45-year-old man is brought to the emergency department complaining of abrupt onset of nausea, vomiting, and headache during dinner at a restaurant. Initial physical exam is notable for flushed face, hypotension, tachycardia, and tachypnea. Further questioning reveals he had been drinking wine with dinner. You suspect that he is taking which medication that contributed to his presentation?

   A. Penicillin

   B. Haloperidol (Haldol)

   C. Clonazepam (Klonopin)

   D. Metronidazole (Flagyl)

   E. Sertraline (Zoloft)

209. A 25-year-old female has a two-month history of sudden and unexpected attacks where she feels her heart beat rapidly, experiences nausea and chest pain, and has difficulty catching her breath. She states that these episodes often occur in public places and she feels the "need to escape" very quickly. These attacks last approximately 15 minutes and then resolve spontaneously, often when the patient finds a quiet, isolated location. The patient denies any significant medical history or substance use. This patient's most likely diagnosis is:

A. Substance abuse

B. Panic disorder

C. Generalized anxiety disorder

D. Cardiac ischemia

E. Obsessive-compulsive disorder

210. A 27-year-old male comes to your office with complaints of fatigue and exercise intolerance. One year ago he had been able to complete a marathon but now can barely run two blocks. He has not been exercising as much, has been losing weight, and has bouts of diarrhea. He also complains that he has started to get numbness and tingling in his legs. He has no other significant medical history, but relates that his hair has recently been turning gray although no one in his family turned gray before 50. The lab reports he has many megaloblastic red cells. On further questioning, you find that five months ago he traveled to Finland to visit relatives and spent two weeks hunting and fishing there. An organism that may be responsible for his illness is:

A. *Taenia solium*

B. *Echinococcus*

C. *Taenia saginata*

D. *Cryptosporidium*

E. *Diphyllobothrium latum*

211. A 45-year-old homeless man presents to your emergency department with a chief complaint of bleeding gums and a cut on his forearm that appears to be healing poorly. Upon further interrogation, you learn that he is an alcoholic and eats mostly hot dogs and little else. Which of the following nutritional deficiencies do you suspect?

A. Thiamine

B. Folate

C. Vitamin C

D. Vitamin D

E. Vitamin A

212. A 72-year-old woman is an inpatient following hip surgery. Because of difficulty with sleeping, she has been given high doses of Benadryl for the past several nights. She developed confusion and disorientation with fluctuating levels of consciousness. At times she becomes combative and difficult to manage behaviorally, all of which are new and out of character for her. You see her as part of a consultation service. The EEG finding most consistent with this condition is:

A. Periodic complexes

B. Diffuse slowing

C. Triphasic waves

D. Spike and wave complexes

E. Theta activity with phase reversal over the right frontal lobe

213. A 20-year-old woman presented to the ER in acute psychosis. Physical exam was notable for green-brown deposits in the patient's corneas, jaundice, hepatomegaly, and resting tremor. Which of the following laboratory results would be most consistent with this patient's diagnosis?

A. Low serum ceruloplasmin levels (<20 ug/dL)

B. High serum ceruloplasmin levels (>100 ug/dL)

C. Low urine copper levels (<15 ug/24 h)

D. Low hepatic tissue copper levels (<1 ug/g of dry liver)

E. Low liver function tests (AST, ALT)

214. A 30-year-old woman is two months postpartum and is breast feeding her infant daughter. She believes that her breast milk production is waning. Which of the following could lead to reduced lactation in this woman?

A. Pregnancy

B. Stress

C. Breast feeding

D. Bromocriptine

E. Thyrotropin-releasing hormone

215. A patient presents to your office with what he believes is an infection. He relates that he has a wound where he cut himself while gardening. Despite treating it with topical antiseptics, it has gotten worse, with drainage at the wound site and nodules that are present halfway up the arm with swelling. The drug of choice for this infection would be:

A. Penicillin G

B. Ciprofloxacin

C. Amphotericin B

D. Metronidazole

E. Potassium iodide

216. A new form of antibiotic targets and destroys prokaryotic mRNA without affecting eukaryotic mRNA. Which of the following differentiates eukaryotic and prokaryotic mRNA, possibly preventing eukaryotic mRNA from degradation by this antibiotic?

A. Eukaryotic mRNA contains a 3′ poly-C tail.

B. Eukaryotic mRNA often codes for many different peptides (is polycistronic).

C. Eukaryotic mRNA contains a 5′ 7-methyl-guanosine cap.

D. Eukaryotic mRNA is translated into protein immediately after transcription.

217. A 23-year-old college student loses his balance while rollerblading and he catches himself with his left palm on the concrete surface. He uses ice and OTC pain relievers to help him cope with the pain. When he sees a family doctor the next day, the wrist pain has gotten worse. The pain is excruciating with dorsiflexion and abduction of the left hand. Tenderness is noticed over the snuff box. What is the most likely structure affected by this injury?

A. Radius

B. Ulnar

C. Pisiform

D. Lunate

E. Scaphoid

218. You are working as a counselor at a suicide prevention hotline service. If you received a call from a member of the populations listed below, which one would be most likely to complete suicide? (completion, not attempt)

A. Married males

B. Divorced females

C. Single females

D. Widowed males

E. Widowed females

219. A 10-year-old female complains of severe headache, photophobia, and stiff neck that began yesterday. Her mother also reports that she ran a fever at home. She is found to have the following laboratory findings on examination of her cerebrospinal fluid:

	Protein	Glucose	Leukocytes	% Polymorphonuclear
Patient	46	79	170	25
Normal	≤30	≥60	0–5	0

What is the most likely etiology?

A. Autoimmune destruction of central nervous system myelin

B. A non-enveloped, positive strand RNA virus

C. Gram-negative diplococci

D. *Mycobacterium tuberculosis*

E. *Coccidioides immitis*

220. A 30-year-old male patient is hospitalized following an auto accident. He has a history of acne, seizures, and hypertension. He suffered a broken jaw and numerous wounds. He was treated with IV antibiotics for wound infection and developed pseudomembranous colitis. Your attending physician tells you to go and educate him about the side effects of the drugs he is taking. Which one of the following side effects would be unlikely?

A. Impotence from taking propranolol for hypertension

B. Sensitivity to sunlight from taking tetracycline for acne

C. Gingival hyperplasia from taking phenytoin for seizures

D. Constipation from taking morphine for a broken jaw

E. Red man syndrome from taking vancomycin for pseudomembranous colitis

221. A 45-year-old man with a history of heartburn has been treated for several years with omeprazole. He is currently asymptomatic. A serum gastrin level is drawn and is found to be elevated. What does the elevated gastrin level likely signify?

A. Zollinger-Ellison syndrome (gastrinoma)

B. Loss of feedback inhibition of gastrin secretion

C. Inborn genetic defect which increases the rate of gastrin secretion

D. Chronically elevated gastric acid secretion

222. As a medical student, you are rotating in the pathology lab. The attending shows you a prepared slide of a liver biopsy. You are to distinguish between necrosis, fatty change, and cirrhosis. You correctly note that the specimen shows steatosis. In the United States, which of the following is the most common cause of steatosis?

A. Anoxia

B. Obesity

C. Diabetes mellitus

D. Alcohol

E. Two large burgers with fries

223. A 40-year-old man develops jaundice while in the hospital following knee replacement surgery. He says this has happened on two previous occasions while in the hospital and resolved without treatment. Laboratory tests reveal a total bilirubin of 10 mg/dL that is almost entirely unconjugated. A blood smear reveals no evidence of hemolysis. Which of the following diagnoses is most likely?

A. Gilbert's syndrome

B. Dubin-Johnson syndrome

C. Rotor syndrome

D. Bile duct obstruction

224. A 25-year-old white male has a weeklong history of grandiose ideas of his own ability, is easily distracted, is irritable, and is sleeping at least 12 to 14 hours a day. Which of the following is least consistent with an episode of mania?

A. Psychosis

B. Pressured speech

C. Flight of ideas

D. Inflated self-esteem

E. Hypersomnolence

225. A 60-year-old black female presents in congestive heart failure. Her past history and laboratory studies do not suggest any renal problem. As part of her treatment regimen, you decide to add a diuretic, and choose one that acts at the proximal convoluted tubule. Which of the following diuretics did you choose?

A. Hydrochlorothiazide

B. Furosemide

C. Spironolactone

D. Mannitol

E. Acetazolamide

226. You are called to see a 27-year-old graduate student who has just returned from a 10-day research trip to South America. She states that she developed abdominal pain and diarrhea on the plane trip back. She characterized the diarrhea as fairly severe and watery, but denies seeing any blood and has been afebrile. The patient states that while in South America, she ate the native foods and was usually provided water by her guides. Which organism is most likely to have been the cause of this patient's gastroenteritis?

A. *Vibrio cholerae*

B. Enterohemorrhagic *E. coli*

C. Enteroinvasive *E. coli*

D. *Shigella dysenteriae*

E. *Clostridium difficile*

227. An obese 37-year-old white female complains of problems with her hands. On history, her hands have been bothering her for the past year. They are worse at night and often wake her up with sensation of "pins and needles" two to three nights a week. She is a smoker, one pack per day for the past 17 years, and gets little physical exercise. Her employment from age 16 to 32 was at a chicken farm on a processing line. For the past five years she has moved to a desk job where she types on a computer more than seven hours per day. Her symptoms bother her often during the day. Nerve conduction tests are indicative of a nerve entrapment syndrome of the median nerve. Where do you expect her numbness to present?

A. Palmar hand, medial aspect

B. Palmar hand, lateral aspect

C. Palmar hand, entire surface

D. Dorsal hand, entire surface

228. Wound healing is a systematic process. Please select the appropriate order of events starting with the earliest:

A. Inflammation, granulation tissue, wound contraction, peak remodeling

B. Inflammation, granulation tissue, peak remodeling, wound contraction

C. Remodeling, inflammation, granulation tissue, wound contraction

D. Inflammation, remodeling, granulation tissue, wound contraction

229. An 8-year-old boy has been complaining of fatigue, thirst, and frequent urination. His family history is noncontributory. One morning, he is found in bed unresponsive and breathing very quickly. He is brought to the emergency room. Initial laboratory tests show the following:

Arterial pH = 6.96; Na = 140 meq/L; K = 5 meq/L; HCO_3- = 5 meq/L; Cl = 105 meq/L.

Which of the following is the most likely diagnosis?

A. Urinary tract infection
B. Diabetic ketoacidosis
C. Gastroenteritis with diarrhea
D. Respiratory acidosis

230. A 44-year-old with man with a history of Crohn's disease comes to your office complaining of another exacerbation. He has taken olsalazine, mesalamine, prednisone, and azathioprine in the past with differing amounts of success. He now states that he is tired of these drugs and the fact that improvement with them was not long lasting. He wants something new. Which of the following agents is a new therapy for inflammatory bowel disease that might be tried in this patient?

A. Abciximab
B. Infliximab
C. Rituximab
D. Sulfasalazine

231. A 36-year-old native of a rural Brazilian village who has recently immigrated to the United States comes to you trying to find help for a problem with his right eye. You see that his eye is mildly injected and the upper eyelid is folded inward. The patient is in a good deal of pain, and there is also some purulent discharge from the eye. Which bacteria is responsible for this person's eye problem?

A. *Chlamydia trachomatis*, serotype D
B. *Chlamydia trachomatis*, serotype L1
C. *Chlamydia psittaci*
D. *Chlamydia pneumoniae*
E. *Chlamydia trachomatis*, serotype A

232. The most common inherited enzyme deficiency of glycolysis leads to hemolytic anemia. This hemolytic anemia is the combined result of reduced rate of glycolysis, inadequate ATP synthesis, and alterations in the red blood cell membrane, causing changes in the shape of the cell and consequently leading to phagocytosis. This reaction is the third irreversible reaction of glycolysis.

The product of chemical reaction immediately preceding the one affected by absence of this enzyme produces:

A. Pyruvate
B. Phosphoenolpyruvate
C. Lactate
D. Malate
E. Fructose-6 phosphate

233. A 26-year-old woman presents to the emergency department stating she suddenly lost the ability to move her legs. When you enter the room, she is doing a crossword puzzle and asks you if you could get her a snack before you get started "with all those questions again." Once you get started and ask her what brings her in, she shrugs her shoulders and explains that suddenly her legs "gave out" and she can no longer move them. She denies any history of trauma and has no significant medical illnesses that she is aware of. She does have a history of depression and anxiety and has been on a "happy pill" for several years. Lab studies and physical examination are unrevealing. You suspect which of the following?

A. Conversion disorder
B. Somatization disorder
C. Hypochondriasis
D. Body dysmorphic disorder
E. Spinal cord lesion

234. A 45-year-old man comes to your office for a physical. As you begin the physical examination, you notice that his right wrist appears to dangle. A thorough physical exam reveals decreased triceps reflex and weak or absent extension of the elbow and wrist on the right side. Which nerve is most likely injured?

A. Ulnar nerve
B. Radial nerve
C. Median nerve
D. Axillary nerve
E. Obturator nerve

235. A full-term baby was delivered vaginally without complications. He does well when transferred to the nursery for observation; however, he becomes jaundiced the next day. The jaundice resolves without any treatment. Which enzyme is most likely to be defective to cause the jaundice?

A. Heme oxygenase
B. Biliverdin reductase
C. UDP-glucuronyltransferase
D. ß-glucuronidase
E. None of the above

236. Bridget, a 38-year-old woman weighting 45 kg, is complaining of new onset pain in her joints. After appropriate history and examination, you decide to prescribe a first-line nonsteroidal anti-inflammatory (NSAID), ibuprofen, 400 mg three times a day. She returns one month later with new onset of abdominal pain and gastritis. You give her a sample set of an NSAID that causes less gastritis. This medication is most likely:

A. Vioxx
B. Aspirin
C. Topical ketoprofen
D. Cortisone
E. A new COX-3 inhibitor

237. A 45-year-old man is injured in a horse-riding accident while working cattle on a ranch. He has a jagged laceration on his thigh. The wound is not cleaned on the ranch but is cleaned and sutured several hours later at a hospital emergency room. A few days later the sutures are dehiscing and the wound is red and angry looking. Which of the following is the most important reason for delay in healing of this wound?

A. Location of injury
B. Type of tissue injured
C. Infection
D. Patient noncompliance
E. Poor management by clinicians

238. An 18-year-old female presents with a two-day history of fever, sore throat, and general malaise. Physical exam reveals a temperature of 101°F. and red-based vesicles over the back of her throat. The likely causative organism the illness is:

A. Coxsackie A virus
B. Coxsackie B virus
C. Varicella
D. Herpes zoster

239. A 65-year-old male with a 40-year pack history of tobacco use has just learned that he is dying from lung cancer. He starts yelling at his doctor, "It's your fault I'm going to die. You should have saved my life!" Which Kübler-Ross stage of dying is being displayed by this patient?

A. Denial
B. Anger
C. Bargaining
D. Grieving
E. Acceptance

240. A 30-year-old man with hypochondriasis and a family history positive for familial hypercholesterolemia decides that he would try to eliminate his risk of developing heart disease by excluding all fats from his diet. His dietary misconceptions resulted in his developing dermatitis, alopecia, and wound-healing deficits. Which of the following acids is likely missing in this man's diet?

A. Acetic acid
B. Capric acid
C. Linoleic acid
D. Formic acid

241. A 43-year-old alcoholic woman presents to the ER with nausea, vomiting, and abdominal pain. On physical exam, she has epigastric tenderness, decreased bowel sound, and a fever of 38.5°C. Laboratory results show elevated amylase and lipase, and abdominal ultrasound shows ductal obstruction. Which pancreatic enzyme is not secreted in an active form?

A. Amylase
B. Secretin
C. Protease
D. Lipase
E. Cholecystokinin

242. A 14-year-old female is being awakened from anesthesia after having her adenoids removed. She becomes excited, agitated, and somewhat combative just before becoming completely aroused. In which stage of anesthesia did this agitation occur?

A. Stage 1
B. Stage 2
C. Stage 3
D. Stage 4
E. Stage 5

243. An 18-year-old Hispanic male with new right upper quadrant abdominal pain has calculi present in the gallbladder by ultrasound. You discover an enlarged spleen, mild normocytic anemia, and elevated reticulocytes. The peripheral smear report references presence of red blood cells (RBCs) without central pallor. Which of the following mechanisms of anemia could be associated with patient's gallbladder problem, in spite of his age?

A. Iron deficiency
B. Folate deficiency
C. Extravascular hemolysis
D. Sickle cell trait
E. Bile salt deficiency

244. A distraught teenaged girl attempted to commit suicide by leaving her car engine running in an enclosed garage. The girl was found unconscious, but in time to be put on high oxygen tension therapy, after which she made a full recovery. What component of the electronic transport chain in this patient was directly blocked by the carbon monoxide gas she inhaled?

A. NADH dehydrogenase
B. Cytochrome a_3
C. Cytochrome b_H
D. Succinate dehydrogenase (complex II)
E. Coenzyme Q

245. A 60-year-old male undergoing chemotherapy for small cell carcinoma of the lung has spiked a fever and become tachycardic and tachypneic. A central line catheter has been in place for several days. The patient's vitals are T 103.5°F, RR 28, HR 110, and BP 100/60. A glance at the latest laboratory values reveals a WBC of 5000/uL, neutrophils 500/ul, platelets of 100,000/uL, BUN 24 mg/dL, creatinine 2 mg/dL. Arterial blood gases show a pH of 7.38, bicarbonate of 16, $PaCO_2$ of 21, and PaO_2 of 55. Urinary output is on the low end of normal. Gram-negative rods were found in the blood cultures. Upon examination you notice a lesion on the palm of the patient's left hand, which you describe to your senior resident as having a black necrotic center with an erythematous margin.

Which of the following is true concerning the organism most likely causing the above septicemia?

A. This organism possesses a toxin that ADP ribosylates Gi (the negative regulator of adenylate cyclase), leading to elevated cAMP within host cells.
B. When grown on MacConkey's agar, its colonies do not form a pink color.
C. It is oxidase negative.
D. All penicillins are ineffective against this organism.
E. It is a facultative anaerobe.

246. A 40-year-old obese male with insulin-dependent diabetes mellitus comes to you complaining of a large, red, tender area on his left thigh that seems to be causing pain in his groin. He states that it appeared the same way as another one that he had previously on his abdomen. Upon further questioning he states that his sugars have been in the 300s. He has managed to lose some weight within the last month. The most likely explanation for this patient's problem is:

A. An allergic reaction
B. Due to a mosquito bite
C. A hernia
D. A result of the weight loss
E. A result of his diabetes

247. A 50-year-old patient comes to your office and tells you that she will be going on a cruise for her 25th anniversary. She is concerned because the last time she was on a boat she became dizzy, fatigued, and nauseated. Which of the following medications would you prescribe to her to start taking one hour before the trip begins?

A. Atropine
B. Scopolamine
C. Ipratropium
D. Dantrolene
E. Physostigmine

248. On your first day of dermatology rotation you see a patient who has a history of fever, headache, myalgias, cough, and rash. She has no sore throat, nausea, vomiting, or diarrhea. She explains that the rash began on her ankles and wrists, then traveled to her soles, palms, and her trunk. You find out that she spent some time recently visiting her family and hiking in the Pocono Mountains in upper Pennsylvania. She states that no other family members have this. You suspect that her disease is caused by:

A. *Rickettsia prowazekii*

B. *Rickettsia rickettsii*

C. A member of the *Paramyxovirus* family

D. *Streptococcus pyogenes*

E. *Staphylococcus aureus*

249. Mrs. Jones is a patient with terminal pancreatic cancer. She has been nauseated and vomiting for weeks and has lost several pounds. Despite the doctor's advice, she takes antiemetics regularly and tries to eat a full meal every hour in order to get her strength back. Which of the following is a stage of dying that she is experiencing?

A. Anger

B. Denial

C. Bargaining

D. Depression

E. Acceptance

250. Which of the following statements is correct regarding the mechanism of action of cocaine?

A. It causes ganglionic stimulation at low doses and ganglionic blockade at high doses.

B. It blocks the reuptake of epinephrine, serotonin, and dopamine into presynaptic terminals.

C. It releases intracellular stores of catecholamines.

D. It blocks adenosine receptors.

E. It inhibits serotonin turnover.

BLOCK V - ANSWER KEY

201-E	214-D	227-B	239-B
202-B	215-E	228-A	240-C
203-D	216-C	229-B	241-C
204-D	217-E	230-B	242-B
205-D	218-D	231-E	243-C
206-A	219-B	232-B	244-B
207-A	220-E	233-A	245-B
208-D	221-B	234-B	246-E
209-B	222-D	235-C	247-B
210-E	223-A	236-A	248-B
211-C	224-E	237-C	249-B
212-B	225-E	238-A	250-B
213-A	226-A		

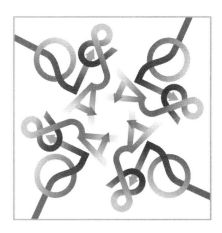

ANSWERS
BLOCK 5

201. E The answer is found by calculating the oxygen content for each patient. The oxygen content (CaO_2) is represented by the equation:

[Hb (g/dL) × 1.34 (mL O_2/gHb)] × SaO_2 (%) + [0.003 (ml O_2/mmHg/dL) × PaO_2 (mmHg)]

If you calculate using the given values, patient E will be found to have the lowest oxygen content at 7.87. You can simplify this equation to Hb × 1.34 × SaO_2 if you understand that the overall amount of oxygen content contributed by the dissolved fraction in plasma is negligible. You can therefore eliminate the part of the equation that is in italics, since it will not affect your answer. This also allows you to completely ignore the column labeled as PaO_2, since a partial pressure of a gas is only exerted when the gas is in the dissolved form. You can further simplify the problem by understanding that each gram of hemoglobin carries 1.34 ml O_2 and therefore the hemoglobin concentration is the most important factor in determining oxygen content. In this problem, the patient with the lowest Hb (g/dL) value will be the most hypoxemic. Hypoxemia is a reduction in PaO_2, SaO_2, or hemoglobin content. The amount of oxygen in the blood, thus oxygen content, is the major determinant of severity. Since PaO_2 and SaO_2 are independent variables of the oxygen content equation, you can quickly rely on Hb concentration as the most influential factor affecting oxygen content.

A. CaO_2 = 8.9
B. CaO_2 = 17.1
C. CaO_2 = 14.1
D. CaO_2 = 15.9

202. B *Clostridium tetani* causes decreased release of GABA from inhibitory neurons. This will result in trismus and spasms of muscles including those of respiration and swallowing. Tetanus is more common in warm months and in areas where animal excrement is prevalent. Although usually there is a wound history or wound on physical examination, this is not always the case. In adults it may have an onset of one to seven days. Like all members of the clostridium family, it is gram positive and anaerobic. Despite widespread vaccination, approximately 60 cases occur per year in the United States.

A. *C. perfringens* is the member of the clostridium family that produces gas gangrene.
C. *C. botulinum*, the member of the family that is the causative agent for botulism, prevents the release of neurotransmitters from neurons resulting in flaccid paralysis.
D. *C. difficile* is associated with the extensive use of antibiotics. It is the causative agent of pseudomembranous colitis.
E. Incorrect

203. D This patient has a classic case of chronic bronchitis, defined as excessive mucus production resulting in a productive cough at least three months out of the year for at least two years. Besides stopping smoking, bronchodilators are the drugs of choice. These patients are treated first with anticholinergics, second with beta-agonists, and last with theophylline. Theophylline is used for nighttime relief. The only treatment regimen that has all three components is choice D.

A. This treatment regimen does not include an anticholinergic. Steroids may be used in the occasional patient but are not first-line therapy in chronic bronchitis.
B. This treatment regimen does not include a beta-agonist or anticholinergic. Cromolyn is used as a preventive in the treatment of asthma.
C. This treatment regimen does not include an anticholinergic.
E. This treatment regimen does not include either an anticholinergic or theophylline. Zileuton is a leukotriene inhibitor and is used in the treatment of asthma.

204. D Delirium is a syndrome that appears over a short period of time (hours to days) where consciousness is clouded; there can be sensory misperception, attention span is shortened, and thinking is disordered. This is common, especially among the elderly, in hospital wards where patients are exposed to an unfamiliar environment, changes in lighting, noises from machines, patients, and staff.

A. Alzheimer's disease is the most common type of dementia; symptoms appear gradually and progressively worsen and include impairment of short- and long-term memory and either aphasia, apraxia, agnosia, or disturbance in executive functioning.

B. The primary features of Parkinson's disease include bradykinesia, resting tremor, rigidity, and postural instability. Fifty percent of patients with Parkinson's disease will develop dementia by the time they reach 85, but it is of a gradual course, not over a few days as in this case.

C. Schizophrenia very rarely presents after middle age and would not show an onset as acute as in this case.

E. Delirium tremens usually occurs two to four days after the last drink of alcohol, not after the two weeks this patient has been hospitalized. Symptoms of the "DTs" include hallucinations, delusions, fever, dehydration, and blood chemistry abnormalities. It has a mortality of up to 15% and is specific to alcohol withdrawal.

205. D Patient's with Sjögren's syndrome often test positive for RF, ANA, and anti SS-A and SS-B. They are also commonly afflicted with other autoimmune disorders, such as Hashimoto's thyroiditis. Symptoms include inflamed, dry eyes (keratoconjunctivitis sicca) and dry mouth (xerostomia).

A. This patient has a positive ANA, often seen in systemic lupus erythematosus, but none of the usual findings. Lupus patients may have a typical butterfly rash over the face, kidney involvement, vasculitis, arthritis, and a myriad of other problems.

B. Although RA can be seen with Sjögren's syndrome, the symptoms and autoimmune panel are more consistent with Sjögren's syndrome. Rheumatoid arthritis is a progressive disease that affects the joints symmetrically, causing thickening of synovial membranes. It has its onset most frequently between the ages of 36 to 50 years of age and is more common in women. The rheumatoid factor (RF) is usually positive, but not always. Morning stiffness and fatigue are common

symptoms. There are tenderness and swelling of two or more joints. Subcutaneous nodules may be seen at pressure points, such as the elbows.

C. Systemic sclerosis is characterized by diffuse inflammation and fibrosis of the skin and viscera.

D. CREST is a mild form of systemic sclerosis. It is characterized by calcinosis, Raynaud's phenomenon, esophageal dysmotility, sclerodactyly, and telangiectasia.

206. A The cystic artery arises from the right hepatic artery approximately 80% of the time.

B. The cystic duct combines with the common hepatic duct to form the common bile duct. The CBD passes through the pancreas and enters the duodenum.

C. Bile is produced in the liver.

D. The gallbladder is not retroperitoneal.

E. The sphincter of Oddi is located just distal to the junction of the CBD and main pancreatic duct in the hepatopancreatic ampulla.

207. A The symptoms and findings in the patient described above are diagnostic for gout. Gout is a form of acute inflammatory monoarticular arthritis. Gout is a disorder of purine metabolism, resulting in depositions of urate (a by-product of purine metabolism) in articular and extra-articular tissues (the classic location of the latter being the pinna of the external ear). Thirty percent of patients with acute gouty arthritis do not have high blood levels of uric acid, which is the case with this patient. In fact, only 10% of patients with hyperuricemia even develop gout.

In this disease phosphorylated fructose builds up, decreasing the amount of free phosphate (Pi) available for the conversion of AMP to ADP and ATP. This increases the degradation of AMP, leading to excess uric acid, and in some patients, gout.

B. One of the mutations responsible for SCID results in a deficiency of adenosine deaminase, which is responsible for deaminating adenosine to form inosine. Inosine is then converted to hypoxanthine by purine nucleoside phosphorylase via a reaction that removes its ribose group.

C. Increased conversion of 5-phosphoribosylamine to IMP, as takes place in some forms of gout, does not result in an overproduction of AMP and GMP. This is because both AMP and GMP can feedback inhibit the conversion of IMP to either nucleotide (they cross-regulate each other's production).

D. During the conversion of 5-phosphoribosylamine to IMP, the entire glycine molecule is incorporated into the structure of IMP.

E. The pyrimidine ring undergoes considerable formation and refinement before being placed upon 5-phosphoribosyl-1-pyrophosphate (PRPP) during pyrimidine synthesis, unlike in purine synthesis where the PRPP molecule itself serves as an early foundation upon which the purine ring is built.

208. D Referred to as a disulfiram reaction, metronidazole is capable of causing the above symptoms that resemble a hangover. Disulfiram (Antabuse) is a drug used for behavioral modification in individuals interested in quitting drinking—alcohol consumption typically results in the unwanted reaction and thus the medication is meant to serve as a deterrent. Inhibition of acetaldehyde dehydrogenase, an enzyme in the metabolism of ethanol, results in an accumulation of acetaldehyde that is responsible for the adverse reaction. It is important, therefore, to warn individuals of this reaction when prescribing metronidazole.

A. Penicillin does not cause a disulfiram reaction.

B. Haloperidol does not cause a disulfiram reaction. When taken with alcohol it may potentiate the depressant effects of alcohol and vice versa.

C. Clonazepam does not cause a disulfiram reaction. The depressant of clonazepam may be potentiated by alcohol.

E. Sertraline does not cause a disulfiram reaction.

209. B Patients with panic disorder experience recurrent and unexpected panic attacks that can involve many symptoms, including palpitations, shortness of breath, nausea, chest pain, and other physical complaints. Patients with panic disorder can also experience agoraphobia, which is a fear of situations where escape can be difficult.

A. Although some of this patient's symptoms could be caused by substance abuse, this patient relates no significant history of substance abuse.

C. Generalized anxiety disorder usually involves multiple worries that patients are often aware of.

D. Cardiac ischemia is unlikely in a female of this age with no significant past medical history. It also does not explain this patient's fear of social situations.

E. Obsessive-compulsive disorder is characterized by recurrent obsessions and compulsions that occupy a large portion of the patient's life.

210. E The patient shows signs of pernicious anemia. Pernicious anemia is caused by a deficiency of B_{12}, which is associated with *Diphyllobothrium latum*. The signs of pernicious anemia are exercise intolerance, a megaloblastic anemia, premature graying of the hair, and neurological signs. In addition, he relates a trip to Scandinavia to hunt and fish where he may have consumed undercooked fish that carry the organism.

A. *Taenia solium* does not have neurological signs and comes from undercooked pork.

B. *Echinococcus* does not have neurological signs and is usually signified in the history as contact with dogs.

C. *Taenia saginata* comes from undercooked beef and has no neurological symptoms.

D. Although *Cryptosporidium* causes diarrhea, it does not cause an anemia.

211. C This patient has the classic presentation of scurvy, a deficiency in vitamin C, or ascorbic acid, with his bleeding gums and a poorly healing wound. His diet consists of alcohol and processed meats. The lack of fruits and vegetables in his diet makes him a prime candidate for scurvy, a disease that prevents the hydroxylation of collagen fibers to strengthen the collagen matrix.

A. Although alcoholics can be thiamine deficient, resulting in a form of dementia known as Wernicke-Korsakoff, it would not be manifested by the bleeding gums and poorly healing wounds but would be shown by mental derangement and megaloblastic anemia.

B. Folate can also be deficient in known alcoholics; however, like thiamine, it would not present in this clinical fashion but as megaloblastic anemia without any mental status changes.

D. Vitamin D deficiency would not present in this clinical fashion, however, deficiency in vitamin D would result in the condition known as rickets, a bending of long bones such as the tibia. This can be present in patients with known renal disease or dietary deficiency.

E. Vitamin A also would not present in this clinical fashion. Vitamin A is necessary for the optical tract as a key component of retinal function. Lack of this vitamin results in night blindness and xerophthalmia.

212. B Delirium, which is very common in elderly hospitalized patients, is characterized by waxing and waning levels of consciousness with an acute onset. There are numerous causes; the one most likely in this case is the anticholinergic medication. These characteristics along with the essential feature that it is reversible if the underlying cause is treated or removed distinguish it from dementia. EEG usually shows diffuse slowing of background activity.

A. Periodic complexes are associated with dementias with myoclonic jerks (subacute sclerosing panencephalitis (SSPE) and Creutzfeldt-Jakob disease).
C. Triphasic waves are seen in hepatic encephalopathy.
D. Spike and wave complexes would suggest seizure activity.
E. This pattern would suggest a cerebral lesion.

213. A Wilson's disease is an inherited defect in copper metabolism, with a resulting accumulation of copper in the body. The disease may present with a neurological picture, often seen as psychosis. Alternately, a patient may present with hepatitis or with both a liver and neurological picture. Kayser-Fleischer rings appear in almost all patients with neurologic involvement. Diagnostic labs include low serum ceruloplasmin (<20 ug/dL), increased urinary copper excretion (>100 ug/24 h), and elevated hepatic copper (>250 ug/g dry liver).

B. The opposite is true.
C. Urine copper will be elevated.
D. Hepatic copper will be elevated.
E. If the liver is involved, liver function tests will reflect hepatitis.

214. D Prolactin is released from the anterior pituitary and is the major hormone responsible for milk production by the breasts. Prolactin secretion is stimulated by pregnancy (due to estrogen), breast feeding, sleep, stress, TRH, and dopamine antagonists. Dopamine, as well as dopamine agonists such as bromocriptine, inhibits prolactin secretion. Other inhibitors of prolactin secretion include somatostatin and prolactin by negative feedback.

A, B, C, and E are all incorrect. See explanation above.

215. E Potassium iodide is the treatment of choice for a *Sporothrix* infection. The history is classic: a wound that occurred while gardening, draining, that does not heal, with an ascending lymphadenopathy. This fungus is found in soil and decaying vegetation, entering the skin by accidental injury. It rarely spreads to bone, lungs, joints, or muscles.

A. The infection is not bacterial in origin.
B. There is little to suggest the wound is infected with gram-negative bacteria.
C. Amphotericin B is too severe a treatment for this rather benign infection. It is not a drug of choice.
D. The history does not suggest a protozoa infection.

216. C

A. Eukaryotic mRNA contains a 3′ poly-adenosine (poly-A) tail.
B. Prokaryotic mRNA is often polycistronic, while eukaryotic mRNA is always monocistronic.
D. Prokaryotic mRNA is translated and transcribed almost simultaneously, while eukaryotic mRNA must first be modified for transport into the cytoplasm.

217. E The scaphoid (navicular) is a boat-shaped bone that articulates proximally with the radius and has a prominent tubercle. It is supplied distally by the palmar carpal branch of the radial artery. The scaphoid is the most frequently fractured carpal bone. Imaging confirms the diagnosis. Prompt diagnosis and treatment are essential to prevent avascular necrosis of the proximal fragment of the scaphoid.

A. The radius articulates with the scaphoid. Fracture of the distal end of the radius (Colles' fracture) is more common in women over the ages of 50 and more likely in those with osteoporosis.
B. The ulnar does not articulate with the scaphoid. It is unlikely to be injured in this case.
C. The pisiform is a small, pea-shaped bone that lies on the palmar surface of the triquetrum. It is not likely to be injured in this patient.
D. The lunate is a moon-shaped bone that articulates proximally with the radius and is broader anteriorly than posteriorly. It is less commonly fractured, but the lunate is the most easily dislocated of all the carpal bones.

218. D Married persons have the lowest suicide rates. Males at all ages commit suicide more frequently than females, at least twice as often, and they tend to use more violent methods (firearms, hanging, jumping). The following suicide rates are approximate and per 100,000.

A. The suicide rate for married males is less than 20.
B. The suicide rate for divorced females is less than 20.
C. The suicide rate of single females is around 10.
E. The suicide rate for widowed females is approximately 10.

219. B The acute onset of symptoms and CSF findings in this girl argue for a viral etiology of her meningitis. Outbreaks of viral meningitis caused by members of the picornavirus occur in the summer and fall each year. All of the major enteroviral groups (Coxsackie A, Coxsackie B, echovirus, and poliovirus) can cause meningitis. Other viral etiologies include arboviruses (WEE, California encephalitis), HSV, EBV, and VZV. Mumps can also cause central nervous system disease and has a winter and spring predominance (in contrast to that of the enteroviruses).

A. Multiple sclerosis (MS) is due to autoimmune destruction of central nervous system myelin.
C. This girl's CSF findings indicate a viral meningitis, not a bacterial etiology. The most likely gram negative diplococci to cause meningitis is *Neisseria meningitidis*, which is also referred to as the meningococcus.
D. Meningitis caused by TB typically shows elevated protein and a decreased glucose on CSF laboratory exam. Clues to this etiology are foreign travel (or recent immigration), lower socioeconomic status, or previous TB infection.
E. The laboratory findings for fungal meningitis are similar to those in TB (answer D). The biggest clue to a fungal etiology is immunocompromise. Fungal meningitis frequently has an insidious onset of a chronic meningitis.

220. E Red man syndrome is from a histamine reaction from too fast of an IV infusion of vancomycin. For pseudomembranous colitis, vancomycin is taken orally. Since vancomycin is not absorbed from the GI tract, it does not cause the systemic side effects as compared to when it is taken IV.

A. Propranolol can cause impotence.
B. Tetracycline can cause sensitivity to sunlight.
C. Phenytoin can cause gingival hyperplasia.
D. Morphine can cause constipation.

221. B Gastrin stimulates secretion of gastric acid, and its release is inhibited by the presence of gastric acid (feedback inhibition). In patients with reduced gastric acid secretion due to powerful antisecretory therapy, gastrin levels will be elevated due to loss of feedback inhibition.

A. Although gastrin levels are elevated in Zollinger-Ellison syndrome, they produce severe ulcers and other symptoms of acid hypersecretion due to loss of feedback inhibition on gastrin production.
C. Inborn errors that increase gastrin secretion have not been characterized, and this patient has another obvious cause for gastrin elevation.
D. In the absence of Zollinger-Ellison syndrome, elevated gastric acid secretion will lead to decreased serum levels of gastrin.

222. D The most common cause of fatty liver is alcohol abuse. The exact mechanism of steatosis is under debate and not entirely clear. Alcohol is by far the major cause of steatosis in the United States and the western world, accounting for more than 85% of such cases.

A. Anoxia has been reported as a minor cause of steatosis.
B. Obesity is one minor cause of steatosis.
C. Both types of diabetes mellitus have been associated with steatosis.
E. There is no documented case of one meal of burgers and fries causing fatty change.

223. A Gilbert's syndrome is an inherited deficit in bilirubin UDP-glucuronosyltransferase activity to levels 10 to 30% of normal. Patients usually have asymptomatic, mild elevations in bilirubin concentration. However, during periods of stress, illness, or hospitalizations, these levels commonly rise.

B. Dubin-Johnson syndrome produces a predominantly conjugated hyperbilirubinemia due to defective biliary excretion.
C. Rotor syndrome, similarly to Dubin-Johnson syndrome, produces a conjugated hyperbilirubinemia.
D. Bile duct obstruction also is expected to lead to a conjugated hyperbilirubinemia.

224. E Manic episodes, diagnostic for bipolar disorder, are characterized by periods of increased energy, decreased sleep and decreased need for sleep, inflated self-esteem, irritability, and distractibility that last for at least four days. Psychotic symptoms may or may not be present.

A. Psychotic symptoms may be present in mania.
B. Pressured speech is common in mania.
C. Disorganized thought processes and flight of ideas are common in mania.
D. Grandiosity, or inflated self-worth or self-esteem, is common in mania.

225. E Acetazolamide, a carbonic anhydrase inhibitor, causes a bicarbonate diuresis at the proximal convoluted tubule.

A. Hydrochlorothiazide, a thiazide diuretic, inhibits sodium and chloride reabsorption at the early segment of the distal convoluted tubule.
B. Furosemide, a loop diuretic, inhibits chloride reabsorption at the thick ascending loop of Henle.

C. Spironolactone, a competitive aldosterone antagonist, inhibits sodium retention at the cortical collecting tubule.
D. Mannitol, an osmotic diuretic, osmotically inhibits sodium and water reabsorption throughout the nephron.

226. A This patient has a moderately severe, watery diarrhea, almost certainly picked up on her trip. *V. cholerae* is known to cause a rapid-onset profuse watery diarrhea, mediated by an enterotoxin. As it is noninvasive, it does not result in blood in the stool or cause fever.

B. As suggested by its name, this organism causes a hemorrhagic colitis, and is often associated with hemolytic-uremic syndrome. One would expect blood in the stool and fever in a patient infected with this organism.
C. This organism causes a bloody, pus-filled diarrhea, and usually a fever, so it is unlikely to be the cause of this patient's illness.
D. *Shigella* causes severe bloody diarrhea. It also usually causes a fever, and the diarrhea has mucus or pus.
E. *C. difficile* is usually associated with diarrhea in hospitalized patients and patients who have taken broad-spectrum antibiotics. The antibiotics wipe out native bacteria allowing *C. difficile* to proliferate and cause pseudomembranous colitis. This patient doesn't fit the typical *C. difficile* presentation.

227. B The median nerve innervates the lateral aspect of the palmar side of the hand. **(See Figure 227.)** Be careful to remember anatomical position, as this is often confusing. The lateral side of the hand is the thumb side.

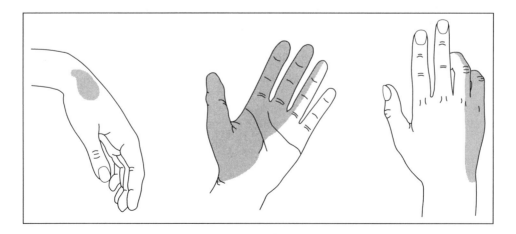

Figure 227

A. The median palmar hand is innervated by the ulnar nerve.

C. The palmar surface of the hand is divided up by the ulnar and median nerves.

D. The dorsal hand's sensory innervation is provided by the radial nerve.

---

228. A The correct order is inflammation, granulation tissue, wound contraction, and peak remodeling. Actually, remodeling starts around the same time as granulation tissue and it can continue for months. Peak remodeling, though, occurs after wound contraction.

B. See above.

C. See above.

D. See above.

---

229. B The laboratory abnormalities are characteristic of a metabolic acidosis with an elevated anion gap, indicating an elevation in organic anions. The anion gap is calculated by subtracting the HCO_3^- and Cl^- from Na, and is normally about 12 meq/L. In this case the anion gap = 30 meq/L (140 − 5 − 105 = 30). Ingestion of organic acids or salicylates, lactic acidosis, and diabetic ketoacidosis are prominent causes of metabolic acidosis with an elevated anion gap.

A. A urinary tract infection is unlikely to cause a severe metabolic acidosis. The patient's frequent urination is explained by the development of diabetes.

C. Severe diarrhea can cause a metabolic acidosis with a normal anion gap, due to loss of bicarbonate in the stool.

D. The patient is tachypneic, which likely indicates compensatory respiratory alkalosis to compensate for a diabetic ketoacidosis.

---

230. B Infliximab (Remicade) is a chimeric monoclonal antibody against tumor necrosis factor (TNF). It acts as an anti-inflammatory agent and has been shown to be very effective in inducing remission in diseases such as Crohn's and rheumatoid arthritis.

A. Abciximab (ReoPro) is an antibody against the GpIIb/IIIa receptor of platelets that is important in platelet aggregation and subsequent coagulation. It is used for anticoagulation in patients treated with angioplasty and stenting. It has no role in inflammatory diseases.

C. Rituximab (Rituxan) is an antibody against the CD20 receptor found on lymphocytes. It is a new therapy used to treat low-grade lymphomas, but has no benefit for patients with Crohn's disease.

D. Sulfasalazine is a compound composed of a sulfa moiety attached to 5-ASA. It is used to treat ulcerative colitis, but is ineffective against Crohn's disease because the drug is not active in the small intestine.

---

231. E This patient has the classic presentation of a trachoma. It is a type of chronic conjuctivitis that occurs in underdeveloped areas of the world. It is characterized by scar traction that pulls the eyelid inward, causing the eyelashes to rub the cornea and result in scarring. Bacterial infections can be superimposed, and blindness develops. Trachoma is the leading cause of preventable blindness in the world, and it is caused by *Chlamydia trachomatis*, serotypes A, B, and C.

A. *Chlamydia* serotypes D–K cause the more common diseases such as inclusion conjuctivitis in infants, cervicitis, and urethritis.

B. Serotypes L1–L3 are responsible for lymphogranuloma venereum, characterized by painless papules or ulceration on the genitals, followed by enlarged inguinal lymph nodes.

C. *Chlamydia psittaci* is an organism carried by birds and can cause an atypical pneumonia in humans.

D. *Chlamydia pneumoniae* also causes atypical pneumonias.

---

232. B Phosphoenolpyruvate (PEP). The most common inherited enzyme deficiency of glycolysis is deficiency of pyruvate kinase (95%). The original reaction involves conversion of previously formed PEP to pyruvate. The reaction immediately prior to it produces PEP from 2-phosphoglycerate.

A. This is incorrect since the question asks for a product of a reaction previous to one involving pyruvate kinase.

C. Lactate refers to the product of the next step, the final product of anaerobic glycolysis in eukaryotic cells.

D. Malate is a product of reduction of oxaloacetate used to traverse mitochondrial membrane in the process of *gluconeogenesis*.

E. Fructose-6-phospate is a product of glucose-6-P conversion during glycolysis, one of the very first steps of the process, and one not directly connected to steps previously discussed.

233. A Conversion disorder is one of the somato-form disorders. It is most common in young women. Symptoms are suggestive of a neurologic or physical disorder but laboratory testing and physical examination are negative. Perhaps the most striking is what is called "la belle indifference" which refers to the matter-of-fact way in which the patient presents, which is inconsistent with the serious symptoms he or she is describing.

B. Somatization disorder requires a variety of complaints in multiple organ systems.

C. Hypochondriasis is a fear of having a serious medical illness in spite of medical reassurance to the contrary.

D. Body dysmorphic disorder is when the patient is convinced that part of their anatomy is deformed (such as a nose).

E. Spinal cord lesion would present with neurologic findings on physical exam.

234. B The radial nerve (C5-C8) controls elbow and wrist extension. Patients typically present with wrist drop. In this patient, this is the most likely etiology.

A. The ulnar nerve (C8-T1) aids in flexion of the wrist and controls the fourth and fifth digits.

C. The median nerve aids in flexion of the wrist and controls the first, second, and third digits and forearm pronation.

D. The axillary nerve controls the deltoid muscles (C5-C6).

E. The obturator nerve is not an upper body motor neuron. It controls hip adduction (L2-L4).

235. C Physiologic jaundice is due to immature hepatic function of newborns to conjugate bilirubin for excretion. The transition of newborns from the womb to the outside environment causes elevation in bilirubin levels and puts more stress on hepatic function. The increased bilirubin level can be due to increased red blood cell volume, decreased red blood cell survival, and increased enterohepatic circulation. Risk factors for developing more severe physiologic jaundice include prematurity, maternal diabetes, traumatic delivery, and an Asian or Native American ancestry. After being taken up into the liver, bilirubin is conjugated with glucuronic acid by UDP-glucuronyltransferase to produce bilirubin glucuronide, a water-soluble form that can be excreted into bile. In newborns, this enzyme may be deficient and allow bilirubin to accumulate.

A. Bilirubin is derived from heme, a product of erythrocyte catabolism by the mononuclear phagocyte system. Heme is first oxidized by heme oxygenase to produce biliverdin.

B. Biliverdin is reduced to bilirubin outside the liver. Because bilirubin is insoluble in aqueous solution, the majority of bilirubin is bound to albumin.

D. Enteric bacteria use ß-glucuronidase to deconjugate bilirubin glucuronides to colorless urobilinogens. The majority of the urobilinogens are excreted in the feces, but some are reabsorbed in the ileum and the colon to be returned to the liver.

E. Incorrect.

236. A Vioxx is one of two (the other being Celebrex) COX-2 inhibitors. Previous NSAIDs inhibited both COX-1 and COX-2. Inhibition of COX-1 can lead to gastritis and ulcers. Although COX-2 inhibitors target COX-2 as the name suggests, they do minimally inhibit COX-1 as well and do cause gastritis, albeit much less than traditional NSAIDs.

B. Aspirin can cause severe gastritis.

C. Topical ketoprofen should not cause any gastritis at all since it is not orally administered.

D. Cortisone is a steroid, not an NSAID.

E. At this point, no COX-3 enzyme has been found.

237. C Infection is the most common and important reason for delayed wound healing. This wound was undoubtedly dirty, and the delay in receiving care made the wound a setup for infection. Sutures in a dirty wound may also increase the likelihood of infection.

A. Location of injury does affect wound healing, particularly if the wounded part is subject to motion.

B. Vascularized tissues heal faster. Tendons, for example, heal slowly because of poor vascularization.

D. Patient noncompliance is certainly a major issue in medicine. Yet, when it comes to wound healing, it doesn't compare to infection.

E. Poor suturing causing tissue necrosis does contribute to poor wound healing. Suturing of obviously dirty wounds such as dog bites may result in infection and poor healing.

238. A Indeed, it is a classic Coxsackie A-associated illness, along with hand-foot-and-mouth disease. In the latter, vesicular rash is found on hands and feet and ulcerations are in the mouth.

B. Coxsackie B viruses cause pleurodynia, myocarditis, and pericarditis. Both types A and B might cause upper respiratory infections, aseptic meningitis, rash, and fever.
C. Varicella (chicken pox) has a diffuse vesicular rash. It has no association with herpangina.
D. Herpes zoster (varicella-zoster or VZV) is an infection associated with latent varicella virus, reactivated commonly during reduced cell-mediated immunity or trauma, causing vesicular skin rash in dermatomal distribution.

239. B The five Kübler-Ross stages of dying include denial, anger, bargaining, grieving, and acceptance. These stages may occur in any order, and more than one stage may present at the same time. During the anger stage, the patient may become upset with their physician and blame them for their fate.

A. During the denial stage, the patient refuses to believe that he or she is dying.
C. During the bargaining stage, the patient may try to make a deal with some higher being in hopes of preventing death.
D. During the grieving stage, the patient may become preoccupied with the idea of dying and become emotionally detached and depressed.
E. During the acceptance stage the patient has come to terms with the idea of dying, ready to accept his or her fate.

240. C The two essential fatty acids in humans are linoleic acid and linolenic acid. A third, arachidonic acid, becomes essential if linoleic acid is not available.

A. Acetic acid is generated in fermentation and can be generated *de novo*.
B. Capric acid, found in large quantities in milk, is not considered essential.
D. Formic acid is generated by ants as a defense mechanism.
E. Acetic acid can be generated *de novo*.

241. C Acute pancreatitis is an inflammatory, autodigestive process of the pancreas. Symptoms vary widely in severity, complications, and prognosis. Causes include gallstones, alcohol, trauma/surgery, medications (e.g., didanosine), metabolic defects (e.g., hypertriglyceridemia and hypercalcemia), infections, and scorpion venom. Intrapancreatic activation of enzymes, i.e., amylase, lipase, and proteases, leads to scarring of the pancreas and complications such as pseudocyst, abscess, and diabetes mellitus.

Proteases include trypsinogen and chymotrypsin. These enzymes are secreted as proenzymes. Trypsinogen is converted to trypsin, its active form, by enterokinase of the duodenal brush border. Trypsin then activates other trypsinogen and chymotrypsin to break down proteins.

A. Amylase digests starch and is secreted in its active form.
B. Secretin, a peptide hormone synthesized in the small intestine and the brain, stimulates the pancreas to secrete bicarbonate.
D. Lipase digests fat and is secreted in its active form.
E. Cholecystokinin, a peptide hormone synthesized in the small intestine, stimulates the contraction of the gallbladder and secretion of digestive enzymes from the pancreas.

242. B Stage 2. Each patient passes through stage 2 when being placed under anesthesia and upon awakening.

A. Stage 1 involves only analgesia.
C. This is the stage where surgery is performed.
D. In stage 4 respiratory and cardiovascular depression occurs. This stage can be life threatening.
E. There are 4 stages of anesthesia.

243. C Extravascular hemolysis is correct. Indeed, at a young age, combination of anemia, gallstones, and splenomegaly should lead you to the diagnosis of extravascular hemolytic anemia. Congenital spherocytosis, in particular, is an autosomal dominant disease with problems forming spectrin, RBC membrane protein. As a result, the surface area of RBCs in these patients is decreased, making them more prone to rupturing during the osmotic fragility test. A central area of pallor in normal RBCs is representative of less-concentrated hemoglobin. This area is absent in spherocytosis. The resultant RBCs are spheroid, making it more difficult for them to pass through the system. They get trapped in splenic sinusoids and are further degraded by macrophages, hence the term extravascular hemolysis. The increased bilirubin precipitates as pigment stones in the gallbladder.

A and B are incorrect as iron deficiency anemia is classically microcytic; folate is macrocytic, and neither of them is a hemolytic anemia. Additionally, they bear no association with cholecystitis or gallstones.

D. Sickle cell disease is the most common hemoglobinopathy in African Americans. It is commonly associated with cholelithiasis (gallbladder stones). However, peripheral smear does not show sickle cells. Also, sickle cell trait does not predispose to either hemolysis or stone formation.

E. Bile salt deficiency is not associated with hemolytic anemia, although it is a common finding in cholecystic disease.

244. B Cytochrome a_3 is the last component of the electron transport chain in oxidative phosphorylation and donates electrons to oxygen to form water. It is the only cytochrome capable of directly interacting with oxygen. This cytochrome can be blocked by carbon monoxide, cyanide, and sodium azide.

A. NADH dehydrogenase forms complex I of the transport chain and is not directly inhibited by carbon monoxide.

C. Cytochrome b_H is blocked by antimycin A.

D. Complex II is not inhibited by carbon monoxide.

E. Coenzyme Q is not directly blocked by carbon monoxide.

245. B The patient described above is experiencing a bacteremia that has progressed to severe sepsis. We know that the organism responsible for this disease state is a gram-negative rod, and we know that there is a strange skin lesion associated with its presence. The description given in the case is classic for ecthyma gangrenosum, a lesion usually caused by *Pseudomonas aeruginosa* septicemia, though it is a rare manifestation. Patients who are in a hospital environment for extended periods of time are at increased risk of becoming infected with this organism, especially if they have an indwelling central venous catheter and neutropenia. This organism is an oxidase positive aerobe that does not ferment lactose. On MacConkey's agar (which will only grow gram-negative organisms), a lactose-fermenting bacterial colony will turn pink (i.e., *E. coli*). One that does not ferment lactose will remain clear, such as is the case with *P. aeruginosa*. Of course, it has endotoxin (a molecule found on the surface of most gram-negative organisms that initiates the inflammatory cascade that ultimately leads to septic shock). It also has exotoxin A, which ADP ribosylates and thereby inactivates eukaryotic elongation factor-2 (EF-2), an essential factor utilized in the translocation step of protein elongation during translation. Thus, it inhibits protein synthesis.

A. Pertussis toxin (made by *Bordetella pertussis*) adds an ADP-ribose to the G-protein responsible for inhibiting adenylate cyclase (Gi), an enzyme that creates the second messenger cAMP from ATP. This inactivates this G-protein, which leads to an accumulation of cAMP.

C. As stated above, this organism is oxidase positive.

D. Although most penicillins are ineffective, there are a few that are first-line treatments against this organism. They include piperacillin, mezlocillin, and ticarcillin.

E. As stated above, this organism is an aerobe.

246. E This patient has cellulitis related to his diabetes. This patient is on insulin and may have acquired a *Staph aureus* infection exacerbated because of the high sugar levels, which allows the bacteria to thrive even more. This patient needs to be admitted and placed on IV antibiotics to control the infection.

A. An allergic reaction would not be limited to one area of his body. We know that he is an insulin-dependent diabetic and he has had a similar lesion before.

B. There is no mention that he has traveled or been anywhere to have gotten a bite.

C. Even though a hernia can cause groin pain it would not cause an erythematous skin lesion.

D. Weight loss would not cause cellulitis.

247. B Scopolamine blocks muscarinic receptors. As such, it is an antispasmodic that reduces activity of the GI tract and is effective against vestibular disturbances such as motion sickness.

A. Atropine also blocks muscarinic receptors, but is not used for motion sickness because of its shorter duration of action and lesser central nervous system effects.

C. Ipratropium is a muscarinic blocker used in treatment of asthma and chronic obstructive pulmonary disease.

D. Dantrolene is a drug used for the treatment of malignant hyperthermia that blocks calcium release from muscles and therefore decreases heat production.

E. Physostigmine is a cholinesterase inhibitor.

248. B This patient has Rocky Mountain spotted fever, which produces a centripetal type of rash in 80% of cases. The etiologic agent is *Rickettsia rickettsii*, an obligate intracellular bacteria. This patient has been bitten by a tick, which acts as the vector and reservoir. Although many small wild animals and dogs carry antibodies to this organism, it is unclear if they are a reservoir.

A. This is the causative organism of epidemic typhus. It causes a centrifugal type of rash starting on the trunk and spreading to the periphery. It is also an obligate intracellular bacteria. The arthropod vector is the human louse.

C. The measles virus is a member of this family. Measles produces a confluent erythematous rash. Patients present with cough, coryza, conjunctivitis with photophobia, and high fever.

D. *Strep pyogenes* is the usual causative agent of impetigo. The lesions are pus producing and that crust over.

E. *Staphylococcus aureus* is implicated in a small number of impetigo cases. It also produces toxic shock syndrome, in which the patient is extremely ill with vomiting, diarrhea, hypotension, and a desquamation of the palms and soles.

249. B During the denial stage the patient refuses to believe that he or she is dying and tries to stop the process.

A. The patient who is dying may become angry at the people around them.

B. The patient who is dying may try to bargain with others or a higher power for health.

D. The patient may become depressed once he or she realizes that he or she is dying.

E. Acceptance is the final stage in the dying process.

250. B Cocaine binds to the reuptake transporter for various catecholamines and prevents their reentry into presynaptic terminals.

A. This is the mechanism of nicotine.

C. This is the mechanism of amphetamines.

D. This is the mechanism of caffeine and other methylxanthines.

E. This is the mechanism of LSD.

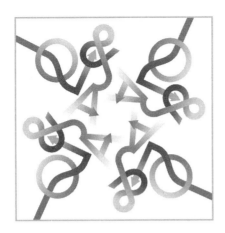

QUESTIONS BLOCK 6

251. A new drug is being developed and tested for eventual marketing. It is currently in Phase 3 of testing. Which of the following is most accurate regarding the process of drug development and testing?

A. The drug is still in the phase of animal testing.

B. Generics of the drug could be available within the next five years.

C. The average time in years to this phase is two years.

D. Efficacy of the drug is being assessed by clinicians after being used in small outpatient populations.

E. A new drug application (NDA) is filed prior to clinical testing phases.

252. A 22-year-old male is involved in a motor vehicle accident in which he sustains a laceration to the posterior medial left ankle. The posterior tibial artery is disrupted on that limb. Which of the following structures is most likely to also be damaged or functioning improperly?

A. Tibialis anterior muscle

B. Lateral plantar nerve

C. Anterior tibial artery

D. Peroneus brevis muscle

E. Superficial peroneal nerve

253. A 17-month-old boy presents with his 10th case of otitis media. He has also suffered from repeated bouts of bacterial rhinitis, bronchitis, and pharyngitis. He is subsequently diagnosed with Bruton's disease (X-linked agammaglobulinemia). Which of the following accurately describes this disease?

A. Germinal centers of lymph nodes and Peyer's patches are hypertrophied due to recurrent infection.

B. Both B and T cell functions are altered.

C. These patients are remarkably resistant to enteroviruses, due to increased T cell activity.

D. This disease always presents with symptoms before 6 months of age.

E. Pre-B cells are found in normal numbers in the bone marrow.

254. A diabetic, obese male with hyperlipidemia is brought to the emergency department by ambulance. The patient is in respiratory distress. He has dyspnea, peripheral edema, jugular venous distention, tachycardia, and a chest x-ray reveals cardiomegaly with redistribution of vessels. **(See Figure 254.)** With respect to the renin-angiotensin-aldosterone system and its role in heart failure, the hormone that directly increases afterload is:

A. Atrial natriuretic peptide

B. Renin

C. Angiotensin II

D. Aldosterone

E. Angiotensin-converting enzyme

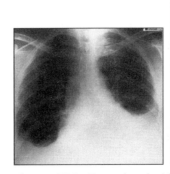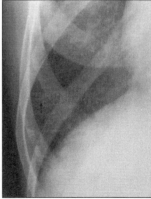

Figure 254 Reproduced with permission from Armstrong. Diagnostic Imaging, 4/e. Blackwell Science, Ltd., 1998.

255. A 23-year-old male was recently diagnosed with schizophrenia. His primary care physician has been using clozapine to treat him for this condition. Which of the following is a possible side effect of this medication that must be closely monitored?

A. Reduced seizure threshold

B. Parkinson-like syndrome

C. Agranulocytosis

D. Neuroleptic malignant syndrome

E. All of the above

256. A 2-day-old infant on your service has begun to vomit every few hours. Upon examination you observe an infant who is hyperventilating and showing signs of lethargy. A few hours later the infant begins to convulse, which is subsequently controlled with anticonvulsants. A CT scan reveals cerebral edema. You begin to consider the possible genetic deficiencies that this infant may be manifesting symptoms of, and order a series of tests. Among other things, blood ammonia levels are increased, blood glutamine is increased, and BUN is decreased. Urinalysis reveals elevated uracil levels. Which of the following enzymes is most likely deficient?

A. Glutamine synthetase

B. Glutaminase

C. Carbamoyl phosphate synthetase (cytoplasmic)

D. Carbamoyl phosphate synthetase (mitochondrial)

E. Ornithine transcarbamoylase

257. A 17-year-old male presents to your office with an infected ingrown toenail. You decide to remove the toenail and inject the toe with 5 cc of a solution of 1% lidocaine. You have used this solution before with great success when you have done skin biopsies. As you begin the procedure the patient screams and states he can still feel everything you are doing. The most likely explanation of why the anesthetic is not working effectively is:

A. The patient is feeling psychogenic pain.

B. There is reduced blood flow around the nail that stops it from being absorbed into the circulation.

C. The patient has a congenital resistance to lidocaine.

D. The increased blood flow around the wound quickly washed the anesthetic away.

E. The tissue environment around the infection is more acidic than normal tissue which inactivates more of the anesthetic.

258. If the RNA from the syncytial respiratory virus is placed inside of the parainfluenza viral capsule, the progeny will:

A. Be fully functional parainfluenza viruses

B. Be synticial respiratory viruses that might lead to croup

C. Cause formation of multinucleated giant cells

D. Be nonfunctional viruses

E. Have parainfluenza viral capsules

259. A 68-year-old man with a history of alcohol dependence is admitted for pancreatitis. While taking his history, you immediately recognize his confusion and disorientation. Physical exam is notable for nystagmus and ataxic gait. What vitamin deficiency is responsible for this patient's current symptoms?

A. Niacin

B. Folate

C. Thiamine

D. Vitamin D

E. Riboflavin

260. A 30-year-old white male comes to your office with the chief complaint of joint pain. After a complete history and physical examination, your differential diagnosis includes ankylosing spondylitis, Reiter's syndrome, psoriatic arthropathy, and rheumatoid arthritis. What initial lab studies would you order?

A. HLA-B27, Rh factor, joint biopsy, fluid aspiration, x-ray

B. Rh factor, x-ray, HLA-B27, fluid aspiration

C. HLA-B27, Rh factor, x-ray

D. Rh factor, x-ray

E. X-ray

261. A 65-year-old male patient is brought to the emergency department by ambulance after complaining of shortness of breath. The patient has a history of hypertension and congestive heart failure for which he is on digitalis, diuretics, and antihypertensives. The patient states his shortness of breath began after eating potato chips and drinking soda all day at a family picnic. The patient is alert and oriented but is pale and has labored breathing with respirations at 24 per minute. Lung sounds are absent in the bases. The patient has a strong but irregular radial pulse at 118. **(See Figure 261.)** What is the patient's cardiac rhythm?

A. Atrial flutter

B. Atrial fibrillation

C. Atrial tachycardia

D. Second degree heart block

E. Paroxysmal supraventricular tachycardia

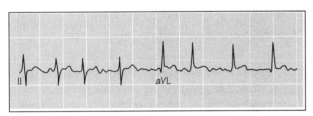

Figure 261   Reproduced with permission from Aaronson. The Cardiovascular System at a Glance. Blackwell Science, Ltd., 1999.

262. A 26-year-old professional cyclist presents to your clinic with numbness of the medial aspect of his palmar hand bilaterally. The numbness is aggravated during his rides and goes away hours after. He is concerned that the feeling in his hand is diminishing and the numbness is bothersome. The likely nerve and site of injury are:

A. Median nerve, carpal tunnel

B. Ulnar nerve, Guyon's canal

C. Radial nerve, impinged between the scaphoid bone and head of the radius

D. C5 cervical root

263. A 30-year-old woman without a history of diabetes presents to your office complaining of sweating, tremor, and palpitations. Laboratory testing reveals elevated insulin levels and hypoglycemia. Levels of C peptide are found to be very low. Which of the following is the most likely diagnosis?

A. Carcinoid syndrome

B. Insulin-secreting pancreatic tumor (insulinoma)

C. Glucagon-secreting pancreatic tumor (glucagonoma)

D. Surreptitious injection of insulin

264. A 5-year-old boy is brought to the ER by his father. The boy was found in the bathroom in a lethargic state with an open prescription bottle of his father's propranolol on the floor. The boy has a heart rate of 50 but is sweating profusely. The initial treatment of the child would include:

A. Protamine sulfate

B. Naloxone

C. Diazepam

D. Ethanol

E. Glucagon

265. A sexually active 21-year-old male comes to the clinic complaining of penile discharge and pain in one knee. A Gram's stain of fresh discharge indicates gram-negative organisms. What infection do you suspect?

A. *Neisseria gonorrhoeae*

B. *Chlamydia trachomatis*

C. *Ureaplasma urealyticum*

D. *Trichomonas vaginalis*

E. *Staphylococcus saprophyticus*

266. A prospective research study is devised to study the adverse effects of smoking. Two populations are identified (smokers and nonsmokers) in their early 20s and the plan is to compare certain measurements of health of the individuals who were "exposed" to the risk factor to the health of the individuals who were not exposed up through age 60. This type of study allows for comparison of incidence rates of a disease in smokers versus the incidence rate of the disease in nonsmokers, a calculation known as:

A. Relative risk

B. Positive predictive value

C. Sensitivity

D. Specificity

E. Odds ratio

267. A 50-year-old otherwise healthy man awoke one night with excruciating pain of his right foot. Over the next few months, these attacks recurred and came to involve his ankles, knees, and wrists, though sparing his hips and shoulders. He also noticed that his right first metatarsophalangeal joint developed a swelling. Aspiration of joint fluid revealed needle-shaped, negatively birefringent crystals. He was acutely treated with NSAIDs and colchicines, then placed on allopurinol. What is the biochemical mechanism of allopurinol's effect?

   A. Blocking proximal renal tubular resorption of uric acid
   B. Causing microtubule depolymerization to inhibit granulocyte migration
   C. Inhibiting prostaglandin synthesis, thereby decreasing pain
   D. Increasing hydration to dilute the concentration of serum uric acid
   E. Competitively inhibiting uric acid synthesis

268. A 78-year-old woman is found on routine physical examination to have an irregularly irregular heart rhythm. EKG reveals atrial fibrillation. Transesophageal echocardiogram reveals a large mural thrombus in the left atrium. Which of the following most directly contributed to clot formation in this patient?

   A. Stasis of blood
   B. Inherited hypercoagulable state
   C. Hyperthyroidism
   D. Hypercholesterolemia

269. Which one of the following classes of antibiotics acts by inhibiting cell wall synthesis?

   A. Aminoglycosides
   B. Tetracyclines
   C. Macrolides
   D. Chloramphenicol
   E. Beta-lactams

270. You obtain an x-ray of a 4-year-old child with characteristic deformity. Vitamin deficiency associated with this deformity is also associated with:

   A. Night blindness
   B. Poor wound healing, gingivitis, and bone pain
   C. Convulsions in infants, microcytic anemia, and seborrheic dermatitis
   D. Osteomalacia in adults
   E. Cardiomyopathy and muscle pain

271. A 12-day-old infant presents with a history of poor feeding, lethargy, and temperature of 38°C. On physical examination the fontanel appears full. Which of the following organisms might you suspect of causing this problem?

   A. Group B streptococci
   B. *Clostridium tetani*
   C. *Streptococcus pneumoniae*
   D. *Haemophilus influenzae* type B
   E. *Neisseria meningitidis*

272. A 50-year-old man presents with a year's history of flat affect, hearing CIA agents talk to him through the walls of his boarding room. He is single and has few friends. He has had difficulty in keeping a job. There is some indication that his thought process has been disordered for some time preceding the past year. Which of the following is associated with the best prognosis in his condition?

   A. Poor employment history
   B. No immediate life stressors
   C. Unmarried
   D. Older age at onset
   E. Slow or gradual onset

273. A 15-year-old boy began noticing muscle cramps after running only short sprints or walking extended distances uphill. He also noted some burgundy-colored urine after these episodes of muscle cramps. Urinalysis revealed the presence of myoglobin in the colored urine. An ischemic stress test revealed a failure of serum lactate to rise during exercise yet ammonia levels were abnormally high. Muscle biopsy revealed a quantitative increase in the amount of skeletal glycogen, though structurally the glycogen appeared to be normal. Which enzyme is most likely defective in this patient?

A. Muscle glycogen phosphorylase

B. Glucose-6-phosphatase

C. Lysosomal alpha-1,4-glucosidase

D. Homogentisic acid oxidase

E. Hypoxanthine-guanine phosphoribosyl transferase

274. A 71-year-old woman who was diagnosed with congestive heart failure three years ago calls you in the office complaining of nausea, vomiting, and "seeing yellow." The patient was also diagnosed with hypothyroidism five years ago, and has severe osteoporosis. Which of the following medications that this patient is taking is the likely cause of her symptoms?

A. Alendronate

B. Digoxin

C. Quinapril

D. Lasix

E. Propranolol

275. A 65-year-old African-American woman presents with back pain following a fall. Radiographs of the lumbar spine show diffuse osteoporosis and a compression fracture of a lumbar vertebra. In addition, this patient suffers from obesity and systemic lupus erythematosus (SLE) treated with multiple courses of prednisone. She takes estrogen as hormone replacement therapy. Which of the following patient characteristics puts her at increased risk for osteoporosis?

A. African-American race

B. Obesity

C. Estrogen replacement

D. Glucocorticoid use

276. An 82-year-old man comes to your office because he had passed out in church. He had been healthy all his life. He attributed the episode to hunger or anxiety. You hear a loud systolic murmur and find an aortic valve narrowing on the ultrasound. Of the following choices, which is most likely this patient's etiology?

A. Rheumatic heart disease

B. Myxomatous degeneration

C. Anatomically normal but calcified valve

D. Dilation of the ascending aorta

E. Marfan's syndrome

277. An elderly gentleman was admitted to the hospital and diagnosed with aspiration pneumonia. He was placed on a course of IV clindamycin. His respiratory function has improved and now is close to baseline, on hospital day #9. On hospital day #8, he developed severe diarrhea and a low-grade fever. On examination, he has a diffusely tender abdomen. Which of the following is most likely to lead to the correct diagnosis?

A. Stool *C. difficile* toxin test

B. Stool ova and parasites

C. Blood cultures

D. Discontinue clindamycin and observe reaction

E. None of the above

278. A 26-year-old man, Josh, is brought to the emergency department by his parents who are concerned about his recent behavior. Two years ago Josh had been in college pursuing a degree in physics but the classwork became increasingly more difficult for him and he began sleeping excessively, withdrawing from his friends and family, and eventually dropped out of school. For the past year their son has lived alone in his apartment and has boarded up the windows and heating vents because he is convinced that the government is sending radio waves into his "energy sphere" in an attempt to control his thoughts and actions. His family has tried to talk him out of this, but Josh remains convinced of this, stating that he can hear these individuals talking about their conspiracy to take control of him. Physical examination, laboratory studies, and head CT are all unremarkable. Which of the following is the most likely diagnosis?

A. Avoidant personality disorder

B. Schizoid personality disorder

C. Schizophrenia

D. Schizophreniform disorder

E. Delusional disorder

279. A infant of Eastern European descent was healthy until 5 months of age, when his parents noted he was making less eye contact and was exhibiting a heightened startle response to surrounding noise. Over the next year, the patient's motor skills declined, and he developed a nonfebrile seizure. On physical exam, the boy was found to have macrocephaly and a funduscopic exam notable for a cherry-red spot in the macula. Which of the following enzymes is most likely defective in this patient?

A. Alpha-galactosidase A
B. Hexosaminidase A
C. Beta-glucocerebrosidase
D. Sphingomyelinase
E. Arylsulfatase A

280. A 79-year-old man presents after stumbling over a curb and breaking his fall with his outstretched hand. He has pain at the wrist with passive range of motion in the hand and pronation/supination of the forearm. **(See Figure 280.)** Which of the following injuries is the most likely?

A. Distal radius fracture
B. Posterior displacement of the distal radius
C. Clavicle fracture
D. Scaphoid fracture
E. Proximal radial head fracture

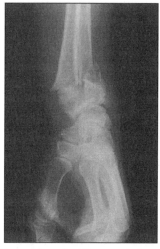

Figure 280 Reproduced with permission from Faiz. Anatomy at a Glance. Blackwell Science, Ltd., 2002.

281. A 32-year-old New York city physician, who works in a community health center serving predominantly urban poor and homeless, converted to PPD positivity on her routine annual PPD test. The year previous, she was PPD negative. A chest x-ray shows consolidation and cavitation in the right upper lobe. **(See Figure 281.)** The patient states that she has had a mild, intermittent, nonproductive cough over the past few weeks. On further questioning, she states that at times she wakes up in the morning wet with sweat, but attributed it to the summer heat. Sputum samples are sent for AFB stain and culture. What is the most appropriate initial therapy for this patient?

A. Wait for the sputum culture to confirm Tb before beginning therapy.
B. Isoniazid
C. Isoniazid + rifampin
D. Rifampin + pyrazinamide
E. Isoniazid + rifampin + pyrazinamide + ethambutol

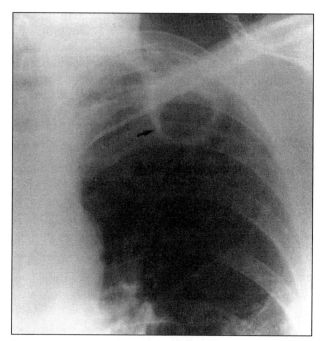

Figure 281 Reproduced with permission from Armstrong. Diagnostic Imaging. Blackwell Science, Inc., 1998.

282. You are seeing a 2-year-old boy with a history of runny nose, cough, and fever of one day's duration. There has been no vomiting or diarrhea. On exam, he has nasal congestion and his left tympanic membrane is dull and very red. Which of the following is the most common cause of this problem?

A. *Staphylococcus aureus*

B. *Streptococcus pneumonia*

C. *E. coli*

D. Mucor species

E. Fungal

283. An 85-year-old man complains of lightheadedness on standing up. An EKG reveals a heart rate of 40 beats/minute and complete heart block. Which of the following indicates the correct order of the conduction pathway of the normal heart?

   A. AV node, SA node, bundle of His, bundle branches, Purkinje fibers

   B. SA node, AV node, bundle of His, bundle branches, Purkinje fibers

   C. SA node, bundle of His, AV node, bundle branches, Purkinje fibers

   D. SA node, Purkinje fibers, AV node, bundle branches, bundle of His

284. Psammoma bodies are concentric, calcified nodules present in several different types of neoplasms. If serial sections of pathology specimens from a tumor were found to be devoid of psammomas, which of the following would be the most likely tentative diagnosis?

   A. Papillary adenocarcinoma of thyroid

   B. Serous papillary cystadenocarcinoma of ovary

   C. Mesothelioma

   D. Squamous cell carcinoma of the skin

   E. Meningioma

285. A 45-year-old busy businessman is referred to your hypertension clinic by his primary doctor. He has been tried on captopril, atenolol, and hydrochlorothiazide with little effect. The patient is overweight, but has no complaints, and wonders what the fuss is about. What is the most appropriate action?

   A. Increase dosage of his current medication.

   B. Combine two hypertensive medications of the same type.

   C. Combine two hypertensive medications of different types.

   D. Instruct patient to monitor his BP five times per day.

   E. Gently and respectfully ask further about his compliance.

286. While on your emergency medicine rotation, a 21-year-old female whose chief complaint is "low blood" (decreased blood pressure) is assigned to you. In addition to hypotension, she is complaining of dizzy spells and new "freckles" in her mouth. Which of the following abnormal lab values would be expected in this patient? **(See Table 286.)**

Table 286

	ACTH	Na	K	Free Cortisol
A.	Increased	Decreased	Decreased	N/A
B.	Increased	Decreased	Increased	N/A
C.	Increased	Increased	Increased	Increased
D.	Decreased	Increased	Decreased	Decreased
E.	Increased	Increased	Decreased	N/A

287. A 30-year-old female was recently arrested for trespassing on a movie star's property. She claimed that the movie star was her husband. Her own husband was called and took her home. What symptom is this woman displaying?

   A. Loose associations

   B. Hallucinations

   C. Delusions

   D. Neologisms

   E. Illusions

288. A 7-day-old boy is brought to the pediatric ER by the EMTs. The baby's mother states that he has not moved his bowels since he left the hospital, 36 hours after birth. On exam, you find him wearing white pajamas with green fluid on the upper half. As you cut off the shirt, you notice a distended abdomen. The rest of the physical reveals a palpable loop of bowel with decreased bowel sounds and an empty rectal vault. His most likely problem is:

   A. Biliary atresia

   B. Functional constipation

   C. Pyloric stenosis

   D. Gastroesophageal reflux disease

   E. Absence of autonomic plexuses in the large intestine

289. A man comes to the clinic whose skin is an orange-yellowish hue. On physical examination he has yellow sclerae and slight abdominal distention. He complains of constant tiredness, has no appetite, and has aches and pains in his joints that started about four to five months ago. He goes on to tell you that he is on no medications, has an occasional drink of alcohol and a cigarette now and then. You also discover that he was injured about two years ago and received blood. Otherwise his past medical history is unremarkable. After completing the physical and receiving lab results (see below) you inform him that he has:

PT/PTT	normal
Anti-HCV	positive
Anti-HBsAg	positive
Anti-HBcIgG	negative
Anti-HBcIgM	negative
HBsAg	negative
HBeAg	negative
AST	markedly increased
ALT	markedly increased

A. Early acute hepatitis B virus and hepatitis C virus

B. Chronic hepatitis B virus healthy carrier

C. Chronic HCV infection with immunization to HBV

D. Chronic hepatitis infective carrier

E. Hepatitis in serology gap (window period)

290. A 25-year-old sexually active nulligravida woman with a history of regular menses comes to your office stating that she thinks she is having another "yeast infection." She is complaining of mild vulvar itching associated with a copious thin white-to-grayish discharge that stains her undergarments and smells like "bad fish." She denies dysuria or dyspareunia. Upon examination the homogeneous vaginal discharge is mildly adherent to the vaginal wall. No discharge is seen coming from the cervix. The area of Bartholin's gland appears normal. There are no apparent lesions on the vulva or cervix. The vaginal pH is measured to be 5.5. A few drops of 10% KOH mixed with the vaginal secretions quickly elicits a "fishy" odor. Wet mount examination is inconclusive.

Which of the following statements concerning this patient's condition is correct?

A. Metronidazole would be an inappropriate treatment for this infection.

B. A marked change in vaginal flora is thought to be responsible for this condition, resulting

in a loss of lactobacilli and an increase in a variety of anaerobes and other bacteria living symbiotically.

C. The organism responsible for this infection is a flagellated protozoan.

D. The organism responsible for this patient's current condition is also a common cause of Bartholin gland infection.

E. Significantly elevated numbers of WBCs would be expected to be seen on wet preparation of the discharge.

291. A 34-year-old white female presents with a history of amenorrhea, excess facial hair, and infertility. A work-up indicated that she was anovulatory. Clomiphene is prescribed to your patient. Clomiphene works to:

A. Suppress LH and FSH, allowing an LH surge and ovulation

B. Block estrogen receptors, allowing progesterone to cause endometrium proliferation

C. Enhance LH and FSH, enhancing the possibility of ovulation

D. Decrease the number of multiple pregnancies

E. Delay the onset of menopause

292. A 25-year-old medical student was told that his skin has recently become yellow. He drinks one to two beers socially at parties and has experimented with illicit drugs in college. At the student center, his physical exam is normal except for mild jaundice. The CBC and liver function tests are normal except that the unconjugated bilirubin level is elevated. What is the most likely diagnosis?

A. Crigler-Najjar syndrome

B. Dubin-Johnson syndrome

C. Rotor syndrome

D. Gilbert syndrome

E. Cholecystitis

293. A 68-year-old male has a history of left arm pain radiating down to his left hand. He states that his hand at times feels numb and other times it feels like pins and needles are being stuck into his hand. He has no chest pain, no shortness of breath, no diaphoresis, and no hoarseness. He has a nonproductive cough. On physical exam he has left subclavicular lymphadenopathy; wheezing, especially on the left side of his chest; and heart: S1, S2, no S3, no S4, no murmur. Chest x-ray shows a mass in the apical portion of the left lung just below the clavicle. This was not seen on chest x-ray taken one year previously. You suspect that he has a type of lung cancer that has been growing for some time. What other findings would you expect in this patient?

A. Cushing's syndrome

B. Horner's syndrome

C. Kartagener's syndrome

D. Carcinoid syndrome

E. Myocardial infarction

294. A 30-year-old man comes to your office with a family history of his father dying at age 40 with a myocardial infarction. Further investigation reveals a high percentage of his relatives on his father's side have died with heart disease at a relatively young age. On physical examination you notice small painless nodules on his Achilles tendons and small yellowish plaques on his eyelids. Which of the following lipid profiles is consistent with his presumed disease? **(See Table 294.)**

Table 294

	LDL	HDL	VLDL	Chylomicrons
A.	Increased	No change	No change	No change
B.	No change	Increased	No change	No change
C.	No change	No change	Increased	No change
D.	Increased	No change	No change	Increased
E.	Increased	Increased	No change	No change

295. A 48-year-old female presents to your office complaining of sharp, burning pain on the right side of her scalp and involving the right pinna. The pain radiates to the posterior of her scalp. "It hurts to move my head and at times I feel out of balance." Past history reveals that she had a cervical laminectomy three months prior to the onset of these symptoms. You prescribe ibupro-fen for pain relief. However, the patient returns the next day complaining that the pain and burning sensation has intensified and that she has an allergic reaction to the medication she started. She now has a vesicular rash affecting only the right side of her face and traveling toward the posterior scalp and within the hair. Your explanation for this rash is:

A. Allergic reaction to ibuprofen

B. Herpes zoster

C. Impetigo

D. EBV

E. Herpes simplex virus type I

296. A 21-year-old male has become progressively withdrawn over the past year, now spending most of his time locked in his room. The year before, he had been a sociable college student, who also worked part-time at a bookstore. Since then, he has dropped out of college and has been fired from his job. He has a flat affect, is poorly groomed, and admits that he has been hearing voices. He is started on clozapine to treat his symptoms. Which of following side effect is of concern when treating someone with this medication?

A. Anticholinergic symptoms

B. Tardive dyskinesia

C. Neuroleptic malignant syndrome

D. Orthostatic hypotension

E. Agranulocytosis

297. A 40-year-old alcoholic presents to your clinic. She would like to stop drinking alcohol. She has a friend taking a medication that makes her sick if she takes a drink. The mechanism of this medication and its side effects are described correctly by which of the following:

A. Blocks the conversion of alcohol to acetaldehyde and causes dizziness, hypothermia, and nausea

B. Blocks the conversion of alcohol to acetaldehyde and causes flushing, tachycardia, and nausea

C. Blocks the conversion of acetaldehyde to acetate and causes flushing, tachycardia, and nausea

D. Blocks the conversion of acetaldehyde to acetate and causes dizziness, hypothermia, and nausea

E. Blocks alcohol dehydrogenase, causing dizziness, hypothermia, and nausea

298. A 38-year-old female comes to the office complaining of fatigue and lack of energy. She cannot lose weight even though she claims she has been dieting and watching what she eats. On further discussion you find out that she is always cold. She also complains of more hair loss than usual, and her skin is always dry. You note that her voice sounds a little hoarse. Physical exam is unremarkable except that her skin is dry and her hair a little coarse.

Labs **(See Table 298):**

From your analysis of her signs and symptoms and the lab results, you inform her that the cause of her fatigue and inability to lose weight is:

A. Diabetes
B. Obesity
C. Hypothyroidism
D. Hyperthyroidism
E. Healthy 38-year-old female

Table 298

Labs:	
WBC:	8.0
Hb:	12.5
Hct:	36.0
Plt:	230
Na:	140
K:	4.5
Cl:	98
CO_2:	29
BUN:	9
Cr:	1.0
Gluc:	98
TSH:	13.5
Free T4:	0.7

299. An 83-year-old black man is admitted to the hospital with pneumonia. He has a high fever and is restless. After a day or two he does not know where he is and seems to lapse in and out of consciousness. He does know who he is. He thinks the IV tubing is chains holding him down. Which of the following is true about his mental state?

A. More common in the elderly and children
B. Cognitive impairment is worse during the day than the night
C. Level of consciousness remains normal
D. Orientation to person, place, and time is usually impaired
E. Develops slowly over time

300. You are taking care of a patient who has arthritis treated with high doses of ibuprofen. You are concerned that she will experience a stomach ulcer. Which of the following drugs has been approved for the prevention of NSAID-induced gastric ulcers?

A. Aluminum-containing antacids
B. Misoprostol
C. Ondansetron
D. Ranitidine
E. Flagyl

BLOCK VI - ANSWER KEY

251-D	264-E	277-A	289-C
252-B	265-A	278-C	290-B
253-E	266-A	279-B	291-C
254-C	267-E	280-A	292-D
255-E	268-A	281-E	293-B
256-E	269-E	282-B	294-A
257-E	270-D	283-B	295-B
258-C	271-A	284-D	296-E
259-C	272-D	285-E	297-C
260-E	273-A	286-B	298-C
261-B	274-B	287-C	299-A
262-B	275-D	288-E	300-B
263-D	276-C		

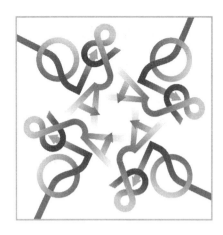

ANSWERS
BLOCK 6

251. D Drug development and testing is a multiphase and lengthy process. Clinical testing (humans) follows animal testing and consists of three phases (followed by Phase 4, which is marketing). Prior to clinical testing, an application for an investigational new drug (IND) is filed. The clinical testing phase, on average, lasts five years.

A. Animal testing precedes clinical testing phases.
B. Generics become available when the patent expires, which would not be less than five years.
C. It generally takes around five years to reach this phase.
E. An NDA is filed during the last part of this phase. An IND application is filed prior to clinical trials.

252. B The lateral plantar nerve is a branch of the tibial nerve. This branching takes place in the medial foot. The tibial nerve is the structure closest to the damaged artery.

A, C, D, and **E** are all incorrect because they are not as near the posterior tibial artery as the tibial nerve. Remember Tom, Dick, and A Very Nervous Harry—Tibialis posterior, Flexor digitorum longus, Posterior tibial artery, Tibial nerve, and Flexor hallucis longus as the anatomy of the posterior medial malleolus.

253. E Bruton's disease is characterized by the failure of pre-B cells to differentiate into B cells in the bone marrow. Patients suffering from Bruton's are very susceptible to recurrent bacterial infections. They are also susceptible to some viruses and protozoa, especially those in the GI tract.

A. These structures are atrophied due to the lack of B cells.
B. T cell function is not affected.
C. These patients are actually more susceptible to enteroviruses.
D. Bruton's typically presents after 6 months of age when maternal Ig is depleted.

254. C This patient is in congestive heart failure. Heart failure causes multiple compensatory mechanisms to become active. These mechanisms attempt to overcome the low cardiac output and elevated filling pressures associated with heart failure. If the low cardiac output is not corrected and allowed to persist, then activation of the renin-angiotensin-aldosterone system becomes prominent. As a result of the low cardiac output, the glomeruli B filtration rate (GFR) decreases, which stimulates the release of renin. Renin converts angiotensinogen to angiotensin I, which is then converted to angiotensin II by angiotensin-converting enzyme (ACE). Angiotensin II is a potent vasoconstrictor that directly increases afterload, causing the already failing heart to work even harder. This results in a vicious paradoxical circle that complicates the problem.

A. ANP is released when there is increased atrial pressure as in found in heart failure. It does not cause an increase in afterload.
B. Renin is increased during heart failure as a result of poor kidney perfusion in order to help stimulate the conversion of angiotensinogen to angiotensin I, which does not directly affect afterload.
D. Aldosterone promotes salt and H_2O retention, further increasing preload but not directly affecting afterload.
E. ACE converts angiotensin I to angiotensin II, but does not itself directly cause an increase in afterload.

255. E Reduced seizure threshold, Parkinsonlike syndrome, agranulocytosis, and neuroleptic malignant syndrome are all possible side effects of the antipsychotic medication clozapine. Other possible side effects include anticholinergic symptoms (which can lead to anticholinergic delirium), hypotension, increased prolactin levels, QT prolongation and other nonspecific electrocardiographic changes, and extrapyramidal symptoms such as dystonia, akathisia, and tardive dyskinesia.

256. E The enzyme deficient in this disease state is ornithine transcarbamoylase, found in the urea cycle. The urea cycle takes place in the liver and is designed to rid the body of excess nitrogen. This nitrogen can enter the liver in the form of amino acids, which are converted to NH_3 and aspartate via reactions catalyzed by aminotransferases. Nitrogen can also enter the liver in the form of NH_3 via the portal blood from the intestine, where it was generated from the conversion of glutamine to glutamate by the enzyme glutaminase. Mitochondrial carbamoyl phosphate synthetase, using 2 ATPs, will then add NH_{4+} to bicarbonate and form carbamoyl phosphate. Ornithine is then added to this molecule by ornithine transcarbamoylase, creating citrulline. Citrulline then crosses into the cytoplasm where a series of reactions (one of which requires aspartate) finally creates urea (which enters the bloodstream and is eliminated in the urine) and ornithine (which crosses back into the mitochondria and enters the urea cycle again). Either of the two mitochondrial enzymes, carbamoyl phosphate or ornithine transcarbamoylase, can be deficient. Unfortunately, both deficiency states produce identical symptoms. These include lethargy, vomiting, hyperventilation, and seizures (due to cerebral edema); elevated blood ammonium ion (hyperammonemia) being the ultimate cause. Laboratory tests are necessary to differentiate the two. Ornithine transcarbamoylase deficiency is characterized by increased uracil and orotic acid levels in the blood and urine. Carbamoyl phosphate synthetase deficiency does not demonstrate this. A deficiency in the ornithine transcarbamoylase causes a buildup of ornithine, and therefore orotic acid, orotic acid being used in pyrimidine synthesis to create uridine monophosphate (UMP, uracil being its base). So, elevated levels of ornithine would also lead to an elevation in the levels of uracil and orotic acid, which can be tested for in the urine. Blood urea nitrogen (BUN) levels will be decreased in both disease states due simply to the fact that urea production itself is decreased in both diseases.

A. This enzyme is a minor contributor to the elimination of nitrogen. It is found in most tissues and catalyzes the conversion of glutamate to glutamine via the addition of NH_3 (from deamination reactions) to glutamate. Glutamine is then free to enter the bloodstream and travel to either the kidney or the intestine, where glutaminase frees the NH_3 again. NH_3 (and thus excess nitrogen) is then free to be excreted as NH_{4+} in the urine in the former, or enter the portal blood in the latter (only to be incorporated into the deficient urea cycle). If the urea cycle is deficient (as would be the case in either of the two disease states discussed above), this pathway will experience increased activity and thereby cause blood levels of glutamine to be elevated.

B. A deficiency in this enzyme would actually result in a decreased nitrogen delivery to the bloodstream.

C. This enzyme is not even involved in the urea cycle. The cytoplasmic form of carbamoyl phosphate synthetase is involved in the pyrimidine pathway, a deficiency of which would not create these symptoms.

D. A deficiency in this enzyme would not cause an elevation in urine uracil levels.

257. E Local anesthetics such as lidocaine work better in more basic environments. In more acidic environments such as those encountered with infection, either more anesthetic has to be used or the anesthetic has to be administered with a buffer.

A. Feelings of pain revolving around minor surgery are commonly not from psychogenic causes.

B. Lidocaine for local anesthetic purposes works at the site of injection and does not need to be absorbed in the circulation.

C. Congenital resistance to lidocaine is reported as less than 0.01%.

D. The blood flow around infected or inflamed tissue is not increased enough to significantly impact the duration of the anesthetic as compared to the acidity of the inflamed tissue.

258. C Changing the capsid around a viral genome is called phenotypic masking. The capsid helps to direct what types of cells the virus will enter into. After that the transcription and translation of the viral genome is responsible for the progeny. In this case more syncytial respiratory viruses will be made. This disease is characterized by syncytial that are multinucleated giant cells (fused epithelial cells).

A. Parainfluenza viruses would not form because the genome is from a syncytial respiratory virus.

B. Syncytial respiratory virus does not lead to croup (laryngotracheobronchitis)—rather parainfluenza viruses do.

D. The viruses would be functional because the genome is intact.

E. The genome would code for the syncytial viral capsid, not the parainfluenza capsid.

259. C Multiple vitamin deficiencies may be seen in alcoholism as a result of poor diet, impaired gut absorption, and altered metabolism. Wernicke encephalopathy is most common in alcoholics and results from thiamine deficiency (due to poor diet). Wernicke presents with a classic triad of mental status changes/confusion, ataxia, and ocular abnormalities.

A. Niacin deficiency results in pellagra.

B. Folate deficiency results in megaloblastic anemia.

D. Vitamin D deficiency results in rickets in children and osteomalacia in adults.

E. Riboflavin deficiency results in angular stomatitis.

260. E One of the key elements a new clinician must remember is not to order a large number of tests upon the initial presentation. This could be extremely expensive and wasteful. Although all the above tests may be necessary at some point, the initial step should be the very inexpensive and useful x-ray.

A. Joint biopsy is rarely necessary for the diagnosis of connective tissue disease.

B. Although HLA-B27 is sensitive for many autoimmune/connective tissue diseases it is not very specific. About 15% of the population is HLA-B27 positive without any signs of autoimmune disease.

C. Fluid aspiration may be warranted if, upon examination, a single joint is hot, painful, and apparently full of fluid.

D. Rh (rheumatoid) factor is an antibody found in most patients with rheumatoid arthritis and is also found in a small percentage of people without RA. You may want to order that test after the x-ray results are known.

261. B Atrial fibrillation is the chaotic firing of many irritable atrial pacemakers in a totally haphazard pattern. There is an absence of P waves since the atria are not depolarizing in an effective wave. All atrial activity on the EKG is depicted as "fibrillatory" waves, or grossly chaotic undulations of the baseline. The QRS complexes appear in an irregular fashion and are <0.12 seconds. The two most important characteristics of atrial fibrillation that make it easily recognizable are there are no discernible P waves and the rhythm is grossly irregular. When the atria are fibrillating the left ventricle becomes less efficient. A loss of atrial systolic contractions impairs left ventricular filling, thus increasing left atrial pressure (LAP). The left ventricular dysfunction also triggers an increase in ventricular rate but at the

expense of increased myocardial oxygen demand, which may increase myocardial ischemia. The increased atrial fluid overload with increased LAP and myocardial ischemia can cause pulmonary edema, triggering the onset of dyspnea. As the pulmonary edema worsens, the alveoli in the lung bases will fill with fluid, preventing the entrance of air at that level and thus causing absent breath sounds on auscultation.

A. Atrial flutter is a fast atrial rhythm usually caused by reentry that gives the P waves a "sawtooth" appearance.

C. Atrial and ventricular rhythms are regular in atrial tachycardia with an atrial rate between 160 and 250 beats per minute. P waves are usually visible and discernible.

D. 2° heart blocks, Type I or Type II, both have an atrial rate that is part of the underlying rhythm. Although in Type II, there will be nonconducted P waves (dropped beats), the P waves are still discernible and with a regular rhythm.

E. PSVT has essentially a regular rhythm with an organized pattern, even when the rate is so fast as to hide the P waves.

262. B Guyon's canal is often a site of impingement with patients who put pressure on their wrists, particularly cyclists. The syndrome is much like carpal tunnel, yet the ulnar nerve is involved.

A. If the lesion were in the median nerve you would expect the paresthesias to occur on the lateral palmar side of the hand.

C. The radial nerve provides sensory innervation to the dorsal side of the hand.

D. The C5 root provides sensation to part of the lateral forearm and provides no sensation to the medial side of the hand.

263. D Insulin is synthesized as proinsulin, which consists of two peptide chains joined by a connecting peptide. Elevated insulin levels and hypoglycemia in the presence of very low C peptide levels strongly suggests exogenous injection of insulin.

A. Although carcinoid tumors may cause these symptoms and on rare occasions secrete insulin, C peptide levels would be normal or elevated.

B. C peptide levels are elevated in most cases of insulinoma.

C. Glucagon-secreting tumors would not lead to hypoglycemia.

264. E Glucagon may used as an antidote to beta-blocker overdoses.

A. Protamine sulfate is the antidote for heparin.

B. Naloxone is the antidote for opioid overdose.

C. Diazepam is the drug of choice for emergency treatment of seizures.

D. Ethanol is the antidote for wood alcohol poisoning.

265. A A very high percentage of sexually active male patients with penile discharge are infected with *Neisseria gonorrhea*. *N. gonorrhea* can also lead to gonococcal sepsis and monoarticular arthritis and dermatitis.

B–E. The remaining bacteria are all possible causes of urethritis but they are not gram-negative diplococci. *Chlamydia* is often present as a copathogen with *Neisseria* in male urethritis and should be tested for.

266. A The study described is a cohort, or prospective, study based on the identification of populations initially free of disease but with a risk factor (smoking in this case) present in one of the populations. Relative risk can only be calculated in prospective studies and provides data on how much more likely a smoker versus a nonsmoker is to get lung cancer, for example.

B. Positive predictive value is the probability of having a condition when the test is positive.

C. Sensitivity is the measure of how well a test can correctly identify the people who truly have disease.

D. Specificity is the measure of how well a test can correctly identify healthy people as being healthy.

E. Odds ratio is calculated for retrospective studies and is an estimate of relative risk.

267. E Allopurinol is a purine analog and so reduces the ability of xanthine oxidase to synthesize uric acid. The metabolite of allopurinol, alloxanthine, also inhibits xanthine oxidase. Note that allopurinol may precipitate acute attacks, so colchicines and NSAIDs are given concurrently.

A. Probenecid and sulfinpyrazone act to inhibit resorption (and promote urinary excretion) of uric acid.

B. Colchicine is a microtubule depolymerizer.

C. NSAIDs inhibit prostaglandin synthesis, responsible for pain. Please note that aspirin is contraindicated in gout because it competes with uric acid for secretion at the proximal tubule.

D. Hydration and avoidance of dehydration or diuretics will help prevent uric acid levels from rising but is not the mechanism of action of allopurinol.

268. A Hypercoagulable states, disruption of the endothelium, and stasis of blood are three potential causes for thrombus formation. In atrial fibrillation, stasis of blood due to poor atrial contraction is thought to be the main reason for thrombus formation.

B. Although an inherited hypercoagulable state may be present, this is likely to have presented earlier in life.

C. Hyperthyroidism does not promote clot formation.

D. Hypercholesterolemia alone does not promote clot formation.

269. E The beta-lactam antibiotics (e.g., penicillin) act by inhibiting cell wall synthesis.

A. The aminoglycosides (such as tobramycin) act by inhibiting protein synthesis at the 30S subunit of the bacterial ribosome. A useful mnemonic for remembering the antibiotics that act by inhibiting bacterial protein synthesis is: "Buy <u>AT</u> 30, <u>CEL</u>(L) at 50." The Aminoglycosides and Tetracyclines act at the 30S subunit and Chloramphenicol, Erythromycin (and other macrolides), and cLindamycin act at the 50S subunit.

B. The tetracyclines act by inhibiting protein synthesis at the 30S subunit of the bacterial ribosome.

C. The macrolides (such as erythromycin) act by inhibiting protein synthesis at the 50S subunit of the bacterial ribosome.

D. Chloramphenicol acts by inhibiting protein synthesis at the 50S subunit of the bacterial ribosome.

270. D Osteomalacia is characteristic of vitamin D deficiency and is an adult parallel of rickets in terms of organs affected. The picture shown here represents rickets. The radiograph demonstrates bowing deformities of both legs, and the detailed view of the right knee shows widening of the metaphyses with ragged, "frayed" margins, characteristic of rickets. The major problem in rickets is that something prevents the normal orderly conversion of cartilage into bone. This is best seen at the ends of the fastest growing bones in the body, i.e., the costochondral junctions of the middle ribs, then the distal femur, the proximal humerus, both ends of the tibia and finally, the distal ulna and radius. The widened growth plate is due to lack of mineralization of the cartilage matrix, and is weaker than a normal growth plate. This may predispose the patient to a "slipped" epiphysis (epiphysiolysis).

If rickets begins in infancy or early childhood, the long bones will show characteristic bowing deformities. The weaker rachitic bone slowly responding to stresses allows bowing of the long bones. Initially these stresses may be due to the child crossing its legs as it sits, and later are predominantly due to the stresses associated with weight bearing. Rickets and osteomalacia are both characterized by an abnormally high ratio of osteoid (inadequately mineralized bone matrix) to mineralized bone, and more than 30 causes or associated diseases have been identified.

A. Night blindness is associated with deficiency of vitamin A. It carries no relationship with bone deformities.

B. Poor wound healing, bone pain, and gingivitis describe scurvy, or vitamin C deficiency. There is no association with bowing of the bones.

C. Convulsions, microcytic anemia, and seborrheic dermatitis are associated with vitamin B6 (pyridoxine) deficiency. Again, there is no relation to bone deformities here.

E. Cardiomyopathy and muscle pain are characteristic of selenium deficiency.

271. A Group B streptococci remain an important cause of neonatal sepsis and meningitis. Maternal carriage of this organism in the birth canal ranges from 1 to 30% (depending upon the population studied and the culture technique employed) and for this reason routine prenatal culture is performed for this organism. Of colonized infants, only 1% become infected. *E. coli* is an important cause of neonatal meningitis as well. *Listeria monocytogenes* is one of the leading causes of neonatal meningitis.

A useful mnemonic for the causes of meningitis in the neonatal and infancy ages is "SEL SIN," corresponding to group B *Strep, E. coli,* and *Listeria* among neonates and *S. pneumoniae, H. influenzae,* and *Neisseria meningitidis* in infants.

B. *Clostridium tetani* is not a cause of neonatal meningitis, but is the etiologic agent of tetanus.

C. *S. pneumoniae* is the leading cause of meningitis in infants aged 6 to 12 months, but is not a leading cause of neonatal meningitis. The incidence, however, is declining due to vaccination.

D. *H. influenzae* type B (Hib) was formerly an important cause of infant (age 6 to 12 months) meningitis, but its incidence is declining due to vaccination efforts. It is not a leading cause of meningitis in the neonatal period.

E. *Neisseria meningitidis* remains an important cause of meningitis in infants, but not in neonates.

272. D Factors associated with better prognosis in schizophrenia include older age of onset, rapid onset, immediate life stressors, being married, and good employment history.

A. Poor employment history is associated with poorer prognosis.

B. Prognosis is better if there are immediate stressors.

C. Being unmarried is associated with a poorer prognosis.

E. Slow onset is associated with poor prognosis.

273. A McArdle's disease is a defect in skeletal muscle glycogen phosphorylase. There is normal synthesis of glycogen, but an inability to break it down as metabolic demands require, resulting in muscle cramps and a failure of serum lactate levels to rise as they would in normal individuals.

B. Glucose-6-phosphatase deficiency is Von Gierke's disease and is characterized by fasting hypoglycemia and increased liver glycogen.

C. Lysosomal alpha-1,4-glucosidase deficiency is Pompe's disease and is characterized by cardiomegaly and increased glycogen stores in multiple tissues.

D. Homogentisic acid oxidase deficiency is a benign disorder that results in alkaptonuria, characterized by dark connective tissue and dark urine.

E. Hypoxanthine-guanine phosphoribosyl transferase deficiency results in a purine salvage defect known as Lesch-Nyhan syndrome.

274. B Digoxin is a drug often used in CHF for its effects as an inotrope. However, it has a narrow therapeutic range, and can cause serious side effects, including headache, nausea, diarrhea, yellow vision, vomiting, and arrhythmias (most commonly paroxysmal atrial tachycardia).

A. Alendronate is a bisphosphonate that is used to treat osteoporosis. It causes a variety of GI side effects, but yellow vision is not caused by alendronate.

C. Quinapril is an ACE inhibitor that is used in CHF. Common side effects include cough, hyperkalemia, and diarrhea. More serious reactions include angioedema, renal failure, and hypotension.

D. Lasix is a loop diuretic used to decrease afterload in CHF. While it can cause digoxin toxicity, by causing hypokalemia, it is not directly responsible for the symptoms of this patient.

E. Propranolol is a beta-blocker used to treat CHF. Its common side effects are bronchospasm, dizziness, fatigue, hypotension, and impotence.

275. D Glucocorticoids such as prednisone are the most common medications contributing to osteoporosis. Anticonvulsants, cytotoxic drugs, and heparin may also contribute to osteoporosis.

A. Caucasian and Asian women are at greater risk for osteoporosis than are African-American women.

B. Thin women are more likely to suffer from osteoporosis than are obese women.

C. Estrogen replacement is protective against osteoporosis.

276. C Anatomically normal but calcified valve is the correct association of a generally healthy 82-year-old with syncopal episode and loud systolic murmur, with aortic stenosis diagnosed by ultrasound. The heart valves are subjected to high repetitive mechanical stress, especially at the hinge points of the cusps, owing to 40 million or more cardiac cycles per year. It is not surprising then to find damage complicated by deposition of calcium phosphate, which as well as a congenitally bicuspid aortic valve, could lead to significant aortic stenosis. Aortic stenosis mnemonic is SAD: syncope, angina, death—sudden.

A. Rheumatic heart disease is most commonly associated with mitral stenosis.

B. Myxomatous degeneration and mitral valve prolapse are commonly cited in mitral insufficiency.

D and E. Dilation of the ascending aorta and Marfan's syndrome, while common with aortic insufficiency, are not associated with aortic stenosis.

277. A *Clostridium difficile* superinfection is known to occur as a result of broad-spectrum antibiotics, such as clindamycin, ampicillin, and cephalosporins. It results in pseudomembranous colitis, causing diarrhea, cramping, and fever. The pathogenesis involves a toxin generated by *C. difficile*, and this can be tested for in the stool to confirm the diagnosis.

B. This is the correct test for a suspected protozoa and helminths. Infection by these agents is unlikely as the patient has been hospitalized for several days.

C. Although blood cultures are necessary in this patient because he has a fever, they will not confirm the suspected diagnosis. *C. difficile* toxin will not be present in the blood, and the bacteria should not be present unless the patient has become bacteremic.

D. Although the patient's GI symptoms may improve with the discontinuation of clindamycin, it is unlikely because the *C. difficile* will still be present. The diagnosis should be confirmed before the clindamycin is discontinued.

E. Incorrect.

278. C Diagnosis of schizophrenia requires at least a month of significant delusions, hallucinations, disorganized speech or behavior, or negative symptoms. However, there must be signs of disturbance for at least six months, which includes impairment in functioning in areas such as work, interpersonal relations, or self-care.

A. Avoidant personality disorder would not include the significant delusions or hallucinations. They avoid others out of fear of rejection.

B. Schizoid personality disorder would not include the significant delusions or hallucinations. They have no interest in having friends.

D. Schizophreniform disorder is diagnosed if the above symptoms have been present for less than six months.

E. Delusional disorder involves nonbizarre delusions (involving situations that could actually occur).

279. B Tay-Sachs disease is due to a deficiency in hexosaminidase A, resulting in an accumulation of lysosomal GM_2-ganglioside. Neurological deficits result, macrocephaly is often noted, and a cherry red spot is seen on the macula. In the Ashkenazi Jewish population, the carrier frequency for a defective hexosaminidase A gene is 1:25. There is currently no treatment and death usually results by 3 years of age.

A. Alpha-galactosidase A deficiency results in lysosomal accumulation of ceramide trihexoside (Fabry's disease). Patients manifest angiokeratomas, corneal opacities, pain crises, and renal failure.

C. Lack of beta-glucocerebrosidase results in Gaucher's disease, characterized by cells with "crinkled paper" cytoplasm (Gaucher's cells).

D. Sphingomyelinase deficiency results in Niemann-Pick disease, characterized by an accumulation of sphingomyelin and cholesterol in cells.

E. Arylsulfatase A deficiency results in metachromic leukodystrophy, where patients develop diffuse dysmyelination within the first decade of life and develop dementia, convulsions, cranial nerve abnormalities, and spasticity. Patients usually die by age 4.

280. A A distal radial fracture (commonly called a Colles fracture) occurs when the radius is broken one to two inches proximal to the wrist. It is common when a fall is broken by the outstretched hand.

B. Posterior displacement of the distal radius is typically more common in children.

C. Clavicular fractures occur most commonly in teenagers and are often the result of direct trauma.

D. Scaphoid fractures occur most commonly in young adults. They are often missed on initial radiographs.

E. Proximal radial head fractures are very rare in outstretched hand injuries unless the elbow is also involved.

281. E This patient very likely has active tuberculosis. Her PPD conversion suggests either latent infection or active infection. The chest x-ray findings of consolidation and cavitation, along with the cough and night sweats, suggest the patient has active disease. For such cases, treatment should begin with the four-drug combination because of the prevalence of multidrug-resistant strains in urban poor populations. Once the culture and sensitivities return, the regimen can be modified.

A. Since this patient's presentation is highly suggestive of active Tb, there is no reason to wait for the microbiological confirmation. Treatment should be started and then modified as necessary.

B. INH is insufficient, even when resistance is not suspected.

C. This combination is effective for pansensitive strains and is given for nine months. However, in a resident of a large urban area exposed to patients in whom resistance is likely, a two-drug regimen is not sufficient.

D. This regimen is not used. INH should be part of any regimen until sensitivities are known.

282. B *Streptococcus pneumoniae* is correct. This is the most common cause of otitis media in children. It is identified on gram stain as gram-positive diplococci (lancet-shaped).

A. *Staphylococcus aureus* is not a common cause of pediatric otitis media.

C. *E. coli* is not a common cause of pediatric otitis media.

D. Mucor species is associated with purulent infections in diabetics and immunocompromised patients, but is not commonly seen in otherwise healthy children.

E. Fungal infection is associated with purulent infections in diabetics and immunocompromised patients, but is not commonly seen in otherwise healthy children.

283. B The electrical signal of the heart begins at the sinoatrial (SA) node and moves to the atrioventricular (AV) node through internodal pathways. (See Figure 283.) It subsequently travels in the bundle of His, separates into right and left bundle branches, and ends in Purkinje fibers of the myocardium. In complete heart block, there are no atrial impulses propagated to the ventricles, and the ventricles often beat at an "escape rhythm" of around 40 beats per minute.

A, C, and D are incorrect, since the order of conduction is as described above.

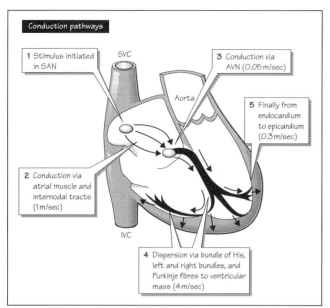

Figure 283 Reproduced with permission from Aaronson. The Cardiovascular System at a Glance. Blackwell Science, Ltd., 1999.

284. D Psammoma bodies represent areas of dystrophic calcification in a lamellated fashion.

A, **B**, **C**, and **E** can all be found to contain psammomas. Only choice D, squamous cell carcinoma, is not associated with these structures.

285. E Noncompliance with medication is the number one reason for persistent hypertension. With further probing, the patient will "confess" to noncompliance with the instructions.

A. Before increasing the medication, you should make sure that the patient is compliant with the medication.
B. Combining two medications with the same mechanism has not been shown to be synergistic.
C. If patient is noncompliant, increasing the number of medications will only enhance the noncompliance since it is more time consuming and difficult to keep track of two medications than one.
D. Instructing the patient to monitor the BP five times per day is unnecessary and he is not likely to comply.

286. B The patient has primary adrenal insufficiency. The typical features from the history and physical are: fatigue, weight loss, decrease in appetite, hypotension, increased buccal and palmar pigmentation, nausea, vomiting, and salt craving. As a result of the failure of the adrenal gland, the body responds by increasing the production of ACTH. The hyponatremia of Addison's disease is primarily caused by a decrease in aldosterone. The hyperkalemia is caused by a combination of the aldosterone deficiency and the decreased glomerular filtration rate caused by low cortisol. Aldosterone is responsible for the increased reabsorption of sodium and the increased secretion of potassium. The random cortisol level is not useful due to the diurnal fluctuations in secretion. A cortisol stimulation test is the preferred test.

A. See above explanation. Patients with Addison's disease (primary adrenal insufficiency) often have elevated potassium.
C. See above explanation. Patients with Addison's disease (primary adrenal insufficiency) often have decreased sodium and free cortisol levels are not helpful in diagnosing adrenal disorders.
D. See above explanation. Patients with Addison's disease (primary adrenal insufficiency) often have elevated ACTH levels and decreased sodium, and free cortisol levels are not helpful in diagnosing adrenal disorders.
E. See above explanation. Patients with Addison's disease (primary adrenal insufficiency) often have elevated potassium and decreased sodium.

287. C Schizophrenia has three phases: prodromal, psychotic, and residual. During the psychotic phase, a patient loses touch with reality and can present with psychotic symptoms such as hallucinations, illusions, delusions, ideas of reference, neologism, loose associations, and tangentiality as well as others. In this scenario, the woman is having delusions or false beliefs not shared by other people. This woman firmly believes that the movie star is her husband, in spite of the obvious proof that this is not true.

A. Loose association is an example of when a person shifts ideas from one topic to another in an unrelated manner.
B. Hallucinations are false sensory perceptions in the absence of external stimuli.
D. Neologisms are the invention of new words. This patient did not create any new words.
E. Illusions are misinterpretations of actual external stimuli.

288. E Hirschsprung's disease is caused by a congenital absence of autonomic plexuses in the intestines, which cause abnormal peristalsis. The resulting obstruction can cause toxic megacolon, which leads to bowel resection. These patients often present shortly after birth with failure to thrive, vomiting, no bowel movements, and abdominal distention.

A. Biliary atresia consists of the complete or partial atresia of the extrahepatic biliary system. Patients will present with jaundice two to three weeks after discharge.

B. Functional constipation refers to the frequency of the bowel movements and consistency of the stool. Ideally, this patient should be defecating after every meal. The stool should be moist and not too large.

C. Pyloric stenosis typically presents at the fourth to sixth week of life as projectile vomiting. The physical exam is remarkable for a mobile "olive" mass in the epigastric region. A barium swallow will show the classic string sign, which is indicative of the narrowed pyloric lumen.

D. Gastroesophageal reflux disease in infants (particularly premature infants) is caused by the immaturity of the esophagus with failure to maintain proper lower esophageal pressures. Most infants resolve spontaneously.

289. C Anti-HCV positive with an increase in the transaminases and a history of blood transfusion confirm that the patient has HCV infection. The anti-HBsAg (IgG) is also positive, which indicates that this patient must have been vaccinated for HBV.

A. The patient does have HCV. HBsAg and HBeAg would be positive in acute HBV.

B. The following would be positive: HBsAg, anti-HBcIgM.

D. Labs would show the following for the chronic hepatitis carrier: HBsAg positive, HBeAg positive, anti-HBcIgM positive.

E. All would be negative except for anti-HBcIgM, which would be positive.

290. B Bacterial vaginosis can be diagnosed if three of the four following criteria are met: (1) a thin homogeneous discharge that tends to adhere to the walls of the vagina, (2) a vaginal pH greater than 4.5, (3) a positive KOH "whiff" test, and (4) presence of "clue" cells on microscopic examination. Criteria 1 through 3 were met in our patient, and although "clue" cells were not seen under the microscope, we have enough evidence to diagnose bacterial vaginosis. This disease is caused by the replacement of normal vaginal flora, which includes lactobacilli, with the following species living symbiotically: *Gardnerella vaginalis*, *Mycoplasma hominis*, and a host of anaerobes including *Bacteroides*, *Peptococcus*, and *Mobiluncus* species. The loss of lactobacilli (which convert vaginal glycogen, glycogen only being present in postpubertal females, to lactic acid) decreases the production of acid within the vagina and raises the pH. Clue cells are often, though not always, seen on wet prep and consist of epithelial cells with numerous coccoid bacteria attached to their surface, making the epithelial cells appear to have indistinct borders and a "ground-glass" cytoplasm.

A. Metronidazole is an appropriate treatment for this condition, though clindamycin is also acceptable.

C. As stated above, this infection is due to an overgrowth of *Gardnerella vaginalis* and a host of anaerobes, not *Trichomonas vaginalis*.

D. Bacterial vaginosis is not responsible for Bartholin gland infections. The most common cause of these infections is, in fact, *Neisseria gonorrhoeae*.

E. Because this is not an inflammatory vaginitis, significantly increased numbers of white blood cells are not seen on wet preparation of the discharge.

291. C This patient is suffering from polycystic ovary syndrome, also known as Stein-Leventhal syndrome. Clomiphene is an antiestrogen that blocks negative feedback on the pituitary, allowing increased release of LH and FSH increasing the likelihood of anovulation. Anovulation is often why a woman with PCOS cannot become pregnant. There are some recent data that glucophage could be used as a first-line treatment in these patients and clomiphene as a second line. Clomiphene increases the chances of multiple pregnancies, albeit a lower chance than with other infertility agents. Clomiphene is not used to delay onset of menopause.

A, B, D, E are incorrect. See above.

292. D Gilbert syndrome is a common and benign congenital liver disorder. The prevalence is 3 to 7% of the adult population, but more frequent in males. The condition is due to decreased activity of the UDP-glucuronyltransferase, so there is unconjugated hyperbilirubinemia with otherwise normal liver function. Hyperbilirubinemia can be mild, chronic, or intermittent.

A. Crigler-Najjar syndrome type I is an autosomal recessive disease characterized with an absent UDP-glucuronyltransferase, which is usually fatal during the neonatal period. Crigler-Najjar syndrome type II is an autosomal dominant disease characterized with a decreased level of activity of UDP-glucuronyltransferase. This disease is generally mild.

B. Dubin-Johnson syndrome is autosomal recessive and the conjugated bilirubin is elevated due to a canalicular membrane-carrier defect causing impaired biliary excretion of bilirubin glucuronides.

C. Rotor syndrome is autosomal recessive and the conjugated bilirubin is elevated due to a decreased hepatic uptake of bilirubin.

E. Cholecystitis is inflammation of the gallbladder. The patient usually presents with nausea, vomiting, and right upper quadrant pain with some referral to the shoulder. Liver function test results are elevated.

293. B This patient has a Pancoast tumor (a bronchogenic carcinoma) that grows slowly and hides under the clavicle when it is small. It is not always detected on chest x-ray. This tumor tends to invade the brachial plexus and/or the cervical plexus, causing pain to occur in the shoulder and down the arm. Because of its invasion of the nerves, the patient may present with Horner's syndrome—anhydrosis, ptosis, meiosis, and ipsilateral enophthalmos.

A. Cushing's syndrome is also seen in the bronchogenic lung carcinomas that produce ACTH causing a paraneoplastic syndrome; it occurs in 3 to 5% of lung carcinomas.

C. Kartagener's syndrome has situs inversus and immotile cilia due to absent or irregular dynein arms within the cilia. Dysfunctional cilia lead to bronchiectasis, sinusitis, and infertility.

D. Carcinoid syndrome arises from tumors that secret serotonin. The symptoms include flushing, diarrhea, sweating, and wheezing. 85% of these tumors arise in the intestine, and 50% of the intestinal tumors arise in the appendix.

E. Myocardial infarction does not fit the signs and symptoms that this patient has even though he has pain with radiation down his left arm. He has no chest pain, diaphoresis, or shortness of breath.

294. A Familial hypercholesterolemia is a genetic disorder that causes a mutation in the LDL receptor and a resulting increase in LDL levels. The HDL level is either normal or decreased, and the VLDL and chylomicron levels are normal. The physical manifestations are the development of xanthomas and vascular disease.

B. The HDL level is either normal or decreased.

C. An isolated elevation in VLDL is consistent with familial hypertriglyceridemia.

D. The LDL is elevated but the chylomicron level is not.

E. An elevation in both LDL and VLDL is consistent with a combined hyperlipidemia.

295. B Herpes zoster is caused by varicella zoster virus that lays dormant in the dorsal root or cranial nerve ganglia. Stress or decreased immune response reactivates the virus and shingles ensues. The rash follows the distribution of the nerve. The rash is vesicular and does not cross the midline. It produces a burning pain and may be somewhat incapacitating.

A. If it were an allergic reaction to the medication the rash would be diffuse and not localized to one portion of the body. It would in all likelihood be pruritic.

C. Impetigo is an acute skin infection caused by *Strep pyogenes* or occasionally by *Staph aureus*. It produces what is described as honey-crusted lesions and is usually not vesicular.

D. EBV does not usually cause any rash.

E. HSV1 is the cause of the recurrent "cold sore" either on the edges of the lip or nose. It may also cause encephalitis.

296. E This patient is suffering from schizophrenia, and pharmacologic agents are the first line of treatment. Clozapine, as well as other "atypical" antipsychotic agents such as risperidone and olanzapine, have fewer extrapyramidal and anticholinergic side effects compared to other antipsychotics. Tardive dyskinesia and neuroleptic malignant syndrome occur more commonly with traditional, high-potency antipsychotic agents such haloperidol. Clozapine may increase the likelihood of hematologic problems such as agranulocytosis, and those who are taking this medication require weekly blood draws to monitor blood cell count.

A. Anticholinergic side effects such as dry mouth, constipation, urinary retention, and blurred vision are more common with traditional, low-potency antipsychotics such as chlorpromazine and thioridazine.

B. Tardive dyskinesia, which is abnormal twisting movements of the tongue, face, and body, occurs more commonly with at least six months of treatment with traditional, high-potency antipsychotics such as haloperidol.

C. Neuroleptic malignant syndrome, which is distinguished by high fever, sweating, increased pulse and blood pressure, and muscular rigidity, occurs more commonly early on in treatment with traditional, high-potency antipsychotics such as haloperidol.

D. Orthostatic hypotension more commonly occurs with traditional, low-potency antipsychotics such as chlorpromazine and thioridazine.

297. C Disulfiram inhibits aldehyde dehydrogenase from converting acetaldehyde to acetate. Acetaldehyde builds up in the blood, resulting in flushing, tachycardia, and nausea. These unpleasant side effects serve as a deterrent to alcohol ingestion.

A. Disulfiram inhibits the second step of ethanol metabolism, not the first. Dizziness and hypothermia are not side effects of disulfiram.

B. Disulfiram inhibits the second step of ethanol metabolism, not the first.

D. Dizziness and hypothermia are not side effects of disulfiram.

E. Alcohol dehydrogenase is the first enzyme in the metabolism of alcohol, not acted upon by disulfiram. Dizziness and hypothermia are not side effects of disulfiram.

298. C This patient has hypothyroidism. Symptoms include fatigue, weakness, cold intolerance, coarse hair and increased hair loss, hoarseness, and dry skin. Lab values show that the pituitary is trying to stimulate the thyroid by producing more and more TSH. However, the thyroid is not responding in producing the T4 hormone since the levels are low.

A. Her glucose levels are within normal limits. This patient does not have any polyuria, polydipsia, polyphagia, or weight loss.

B. Obesity does not cause any of the symptoms that this patient is experiencing.

D. Hyperthyroidism causes fatigue but the patient also experiences the following: lid lag, stare, weakness of eye muscles, exophthalmus, pretibial myxedema, nervousness, palpitations, weight loss, and brittle nails. Lab values show an elevated free T4 and decreased TSH. There is often an enlarged thyroid on exam.

E. This patient has hypothyroidism and is not healthy.

299. A This elderly man is suffering from delirium. Delirium often develops in young children and the elderly, and often occurs in unfamiliar settings.

B. Cognitive impairment is often worse in the early morning and the night.

C. The level of consciousness is impaired in delirium, and is often normal in dementia.

D. Orientation to person often remains intact in delirium.

E. Unlike dementia, delirium often develops suddenly.

300. B Misoprostol is an analog of prostaglandin E1. Prostaglandins stimulate the production of bicarbonate and mucus, thereby helping to prevent the erosive effects on the gastric mucosa that NSAIDs cause.

A. Aluminum-containing antacids are not approved for NSAID prophylaxis.

C. This is an antinausea medication.

D. This is a histamine receptor blocker not approved for NSAID prophylaxis.

E. This is an antianaerobe and antiprotozoal medication.

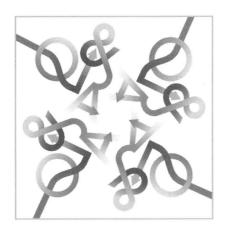

QUESTIONS
BLOCK 7

301. A 68-year-old male nursing home patient who is confined to a wheelchair complains of left leg tenderness. Your physical examination reveals acute calf tenderness and warmth to palpation. The left extremity is red and superficial veins are visible. Doppler ultrasound confirms your suspicion and you begin treatment with heparin therapy. In relation to the cascade of events during blood coagulation, the activity of which regulatory protein is stimulated by heparin?

A. Plasmin
B. Plasminogen
C. Antithrombin III
D. Prothrombin
E. Factor VII

302. A 23-year-old male has an eight-month history of staying inside his apartment because he believes the FBI is after him and they will shoot him if he goes outside. He often hears voices coming from his television that tell him not to answer the phone and to hide in his apartment. He occasionally dresses inappropriately and his speech is frequently disorganized. He has been unable to hold a steady job for the past six months. Which of the following medications would be an appropriate treatment option for this patient?

A. Sertraline
B. Methylphenidate
C. Lithium
D. Citalopram
E. Clozapine

303. A 25-year-old patient comes to the emergency room with a stab wound in the abdomen. On day 7 of his hospital stay he goes into acute shock. Pus is seeping from the stab wound and he is febrile. He is given medication to stabilize the blood pressure and then a biopsy is done of the wound. A gram-positive, coagulase-positive organism is grown out from the biopsy. The most likely causative agent:

A. Also can cause food poisoning
B. Is mostly commonly associated with prosthetic infections
C. Can also lead to scarlet fever
D. Is a major cause of meningitis
E. Is a leading cause of sexually transmitted disease

304. A 65-year-old woman presents to the hospital with fever and a debilitated appearance. She has a history of recurrent urinary tract infections. A urine culture grows a *Pseudomonas* species, with a colony count >100,000. Which bactericidal antibiotic would be appropriate to treat her with?

A. Erythromycin
B. Tobramycin
C. Tetracycline
D. Trimethoprim
E. Sulfamethoxazole

305. An 18-year-old male is involved in a bike accident. He fell from the bike and broke his fall with an outstretched left arm. He now complains of numbness in the medial $1\frac{1}{2}$ fingers and general weakness in moving his fingers and thumb. Sensation in the hand and arm is otherwise grossly intact. The lesion is in which of the following nerves?

A. Musculocutaneous
B. Median
C. Ulnar
D. Radial
E. Long thoracic

306. A 19-year-old female college student presents to the student health clinic complaining of a one-week history of fever, fatigue, sore throat, and dysphagia. She was found to have splenomegaly, diffuse lymphadenopathy in the neck, and 3+ swollen tonsils with white exudate. She took amoxicillin and developed a diffuse abdominal rash. She is most likely suffering from:

A. HIV

B. Infectious mononucleosis

C. Hodgkin's lymphoma

D. Streptococcal pharyngitis

E. Non-Hodgkin's lymphoma

307. A 6-year-old African-American male presents to your clinic with symptoms of pneumonia. His mother complains that he has constantly been getting sick ever since he was 1 year old; most illnesses were treated and relieved with antibiotics. He also complains of sharp pains in his knee joints and a poor tolerance for exercise. As his doctor, you suspect sickle cell anemia. Which of the following tests would be most accurate for this diagnosis?

A. Polymerase chain reaction (PCR)

B. Betke-Kleihauer acid elution test

C. X-ray crystallography

D. Sanger DNA chain termination method

E. Gel electrophoresis

308. A 55-year-old man is admitted to the hospital with a large abscess on his right arm. After drainage of the abscess, the culture comes back as *Staph aureus*, which is resistant to penicillin G but sensitive to methicillin. The patient has had prior kidney problems. The physician in charge would most likely choose:

A. Ampicillin

B. Ticarcillin

C. Penicillin V

D. Oxacillin

E. Nafcillin

309. A 25-year-old male was an unrestrained driver of a pickup truck that collided with a concrete wall at high speed. The patient is diaphoretic with a weak, rapid, and irregular pulse of 140 beats per minute. The blood pressure is now 82/60 and you notice jugular venous distention. The patient's lungs are

clear to auscultation but the heart sounds are muffled. The patient is suffering from cardiac tamponade. **(See Figure 309.)** A change in which wave of the jugular venous pulse best reflects this condition?

A. A-wave

B. C-wave

C. T-wave

D. V-wave

E. Y-descent

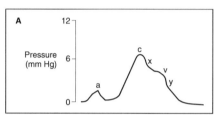

Figure 309   Reproduced with permission from Ayala. Pathophysiology for the Boards and Wards. Blackwell Science, Inc., 2000.

310. The following is an oxygen-hemoglobin dissociation curve for a healthy 25-year-old male. **(See Figure 310.)** Which of the following would decrease affinity of hemoglobin for oxygen (i.e., cause a right shift of the curve)?

A. Decreased temperature

B. Decreased 2,3-DPG concentration

C. Hemoglobin F

D. Exercise

E. Carbon monoxide poisoning

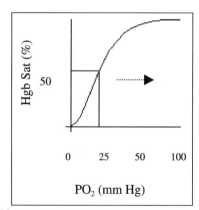

Figure 310

311. A 50-year-old white male presents to your emergency department with a chief complaint of chest pain radiating down to his left arm and up into his chin. You immediately obtain an ECG which shows acute ST segment elevation suggestive of acute myocardial infarction. Which of the following laboratory studies could be immediately obtained that would support this diagnosis early (within 24 to 36 hours)?

A. CK-MB

B. CK-BB

C. CK-MM

D. LDH

E. None of the above

312. A child is born and develops herpes encephalitis. The causative agent is:

A. An enveloped, single-strand DNA virus

B. An enveloped, double-strand DNA virus

C. An enveloped DNA virus with a circular genome that is largely double-stranded

D. A non-enveloped, single-strand DNA virus

E. A non-enveloped, double-stranded DNA virus

F. An enveloped, positive-strand RNA virus that replicates via a DNA intermediate

313. In order to perform a carotid endarterectomy on a patient, a new procedure is developed that allows the surgeon to clamp the external carotid artery just after it forms from the bifurcation of the common carotid artery. **(See Figure 313.)** If the external carotid artery is clamped at its origin, which artery would be nearest to this obstruction?

A. Inferior thyroid artery

B. Superior thyroid artery

C. Lingual artery

D. Vertebral artery

E. Facial artery

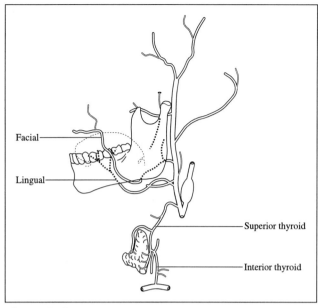

Figure 313

314. A 25-year-old white male is undergoing surgery for appendicitis. He has never had major surgery before and there is no apparent family history of problems related to surgery. He is administered an induction agent, followed by an inhalation anesthetic gas. His temperature rises rapidly to 106°F. Which of the following drugs should be administered?

A. Dantrolene

B. Succinylcholine

C. Propranolol

D. Acetaminophen

E. Halothane

315. A 50-year-old man presents to your clinic complaining of fatigue with exertion. Previously, he was able to walk several miles without difficulty, and now he tires after walking just a few blocks. He has a history of chronic atrophic gastritis, confirmed by endoscopic biopsy several years ago. He takes a multivitamin daily and eats a regular diet that includes leafy vegetables. He denies excessive alcohol use. A CBC reveals a hematocrit of 28% with an MCV of 110 μm^3. Deficiency of which of the following vitamins is responsible for this patient's anemia?

A. Folic acid

B. Niacin

C. Vitamin B12

D. Vitamin C

316. A 9-month-old girl is referred because of mental retardation, a large head, and loss of motor skills. Examination reveals a cherry red spot on each retina. Which of the following organelle functions is defective in this disease?

    A. Lysosomal storage

    B. Mitochondrial ATP production

    C. Ribosomal protein synthesis

    D. Nuclear transcription of DNA to mRNA

317. A 28-year-old man presents to his dentist complaining of a broken tooth incurred in a fight with a stranger. He is recently out of jail where he spent time for burglary and forgery charges (the patient shares this rather proudly), and has a history of "behavior problems" dating back to early childhood. Which of the following diagnoses is most likely given this history?

    A. Malingering

    B. Antisocial personality disorder

    C. Dependent personality disorder

    D. Conversion disorder

    E. Conduct disorder

318. A physician places a patient on an experimental antiseizure medication. Two weeks after starting the medication, routine screening reveals the patient's plasma level of the medication is 9 mg/L. The therapeutic plasma level for the medication is 1 to 1.5 mg/L and the plasma $t_{1/2}$ for the medication is 1.3 days. How long should this medication be withheld for the plasma level to fall within the therapeutic range?

    A. 0 days

    B. 1.3 days

    C. 2.6 days

    D. 3.9 days

    E. 5.2 days

319. A 70-year-old male smoker presents to the ER with an eight-day history of dyspnea and cough. Studies reveal a large mass in the right mainstem bronchus that is found on biopsy to be a squamous cell carcinoma. This cancer:

    A. Usually metastasizes earlier than small cell cancers

    B. Tends to develop in the periphery of the lung

    C. Rarely metastasizes to the brain

    D. Commonly results in hypercalcemia

    E. Develops from Kulchitsky cells

320. As you walk in to the pantry to grab some more canned yams, a rat runs out from behind the potatoes. Startled, you let out a shriek. What is the appropriate autonomic nervous system response?

    A. Dilation of the pupils, increased heart rate, decreased gastrointestinal blood flow, dilation of the bronchial tubes

    B. Constriction of the pupils, increased heart rate, decreased gastrointestinal blood flow, constriction of the bronchial tubes

    C. Constriction of the pupils, increased heart rate, increased gastrointestinal blood flow, dilation of the bronchial tubes

    D. Dilation of the pupils, decreased heart rate, increased gastrointestinal blood flow, constriction of the bronchial tubes

    E. Constriction of the pupils, decreased heart rate, increased gastrointestinal blood flow, dilation of the bronchial tubes

321. A 35-year-old woman presents to your clinic with a complaint of headache and weakness. Her blood pressure one year ago was 120/80 mm Hg; it is currently 160/105 mm Hg. She is not taking any medications. Physical exam reveals a thin woman with normal body habitus, and is otherwise remarkable only for elevated blood pressure. A metabolic panel reveals the following values:

Na = 147, K = 2.3, Cl = 96, $HCO_3^- = 41$

Which of the following is the most likely diagnosis?

    A. Primary hyperaldosteronism (Conn's syndrome)

    B. Cushing's syndrome

    C. Adrenocortical insufficiency (Addison's disease)

    D. High dietary intake of sodium chloride

322. A 35-year-old woman comes into the ER with severe right-sided flank pain that has been present for about one day. She is afebrile and vital signs are stable. On exam, the patient has severe right CVA tenderness. When asked about dysuria or hematuria, the patient denies such symptoms at the present time. However, she states she has had numerous episodes of pain and burning on urination in the past two years. She has never gone to the doctor for these, and they eventually resolve. Renal ultrasound shows a large calculus in the renal pelvis of the right kidney. (**See Figure 322.**) Which organism was most likely causing the patient's previous UTIs?

    A. *Escherichia coli*

    B. *Candida albicans*

C. *Staphylococcus aureus*

D. *Klebsiella pneumoniae*

E. *Proteus mirabilis*

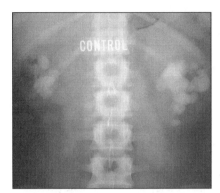

Figure 322 Reproduced with permission from Axford. Medicine. Blackwell Science, Ltd., 1996.

323. A 46-year-old man comes into the ER complaining of generalized weakness. He denies chest pain or palpitations, but the EKG shows diffuse, flattened T waves and prominent U waves. The patient has a history of hypertension, but cannot remember which agent he takes for this condition. You send a blood specimen to the laboratory, suspecting an electrolyte disorder. **(See Figure 323.)** Which of the following drugs could have caused the suspected electrolyte imbalance?

A. Monopril

B. Spironolactone

C. Amiloride

D. Irbesartan

E. Furosemide

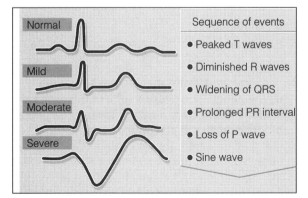

Figure 323 Reproduced with permission from Axford. Medicine. Blackwell Science, Ltd., 1996.

324. A 15-year-old female with type I diabetes mellitus presents to the emergency room. She informs you that she has not been taking her insulin for several days, because she had "the flu" and was not eating very much. On examination, she is feverish and her heart and respiratory rates are increased. Her breath has a peculiar, fruity odor, and her mucous membranes are dry. Laboratory testing confirms elevated blood glucose and a metabolic acidosis. Which of the following molecules is likely present at high levels in her plasma?

A. Ascorbic acid

B. Folic acid

C. β-hydroxybutyrate

D. Oxaloacetate

325. In which of the following conditions is the prevalence most likely to exceed incidence?

A. Chickenpox

B. Mononucleosis

C. Diabetes

D. Gastroenteritis

E. Influenza

326. An 8-year-old girl is brought to your clinic by her mother. Seven days ago, she was skateboarding with a group of friends when the skateboard shot out from under one of the boys and hit her daughter in the left lower leg. On exam, she has a large ecchymosis on the lateral aspect of her knee near the head of the fibula. She is unable to dorsiflex or evert her left foot and her ankle jerk is intact. Which of the following is the most likely mechanism of her injury?

A. Avascular necrosis of the left femoral head

B. Injury to L4-S4

C. Ischemia to the tibial nerve

D. Defect in the dorsal vertebral arches

E. Tissue swelling and inflammation

327. A 69-year-old woman with a history of congestive heart failure is found to be in atrial fibrillation while in the hospital. She has been placed on Coumadin to prevent any thrombus formation. Which of the following drugs can be used to pharmacologically convert the patient back to sinus rhythm?

   A. Procainamide

   B. Atenolol

   C. Diltiazem

   D. Digoxin

   E. Verapamil

328. A 25-year-old man reports a history of "dozens" of skin cancers having been removed from sun-exposed areas on his forehead, face, arms, and hands. He has also had telangiectases, freckles, and keratoses. One of his four siblings is similarly affected, along with some other relatives. Examination reveals very dry, pigmented skin and tumors on his eyelids. Which of the following genetic defects likely accounts for this disease?

   A. Defective recognition and repair of damaged DNA

   B. Defective immune system that fails to destroy skin cancers

   C. Deficiency of the enzyme tyrosinase

   D. Deficiency of hypoxanthine-guanine phosphoribosyl transferase (HGPRT)

329. An 82-year-old white female nursing home resident presents with a history of a painful left lower jaw and foul taste on that side of her mouth for about one week. She now has a fever of 102°F, cough, and chest pain. An abscess in one lung is diagnosed. The most likely organism linking both is:

   A. *Strep mutans*

   B. *Eikenella corrodens*

   C. *Actinomyces israelii*

   D. *Candida*

   E. *Staph aureus*

330. A 39-year-old woman develops chest tightness after watching TV, and the discomfort radiates to the neck and left arm. The symptoms go away after a few minutes. She has no significant medical history, and her family history is noncontributory. Assuming that her coronary artery had suffered a spasm and reduced the diameter to half,

what would be the resistance of the vessel compared to when it is healthy?

   A. 16x

   B. 8x

   C. 4x

   D. 1/4x

   E. 1/8x

   F. 1/16x

331. A child of Ashkenazi Jewish descent began to exhibit motor incoordination that quickly progressed to seizures and mental decline. He has coarse facies and is discovered to have a foveal cherry red spot on ophthalmologic examination. He is diagnosed with Tay-Sachs disease, which has a prevalence of 1:2000 in the Ashkenazi Jewish population. The etiology of this disease involves the lysosomal accumulation of gangliosides due to a splice site mutation, or frameshift mutation with stop codon on the long arm of chromosome 15. This results in which reduced or absent enzyme?

   A. Alpha-1,4-glucosidase

   B. Hexosaminidase-A

   C. Alpha-galactosidase A

   D. Sphingomyelinase

   E. Arylsulfatase A

332. A 5-year-old child is brought into the doctor's office for treatment of persistent bed-wetting. If you were to do a sleep study on this child, what types of EEG waves would most likely be present when the bed-wetting event occurs?

   A. Sleep spindles and K complexes

   B. Delta waves

   C. Beta waves, sawtooth in appearance

   D. Theta waves

   E. Alpha waves

333. A 45-year-old white man comes to your office as a new patient. He needs a refill of one of his medications which he ran out of several days ago, "a blood pressure medication," but doesn't recall the specific name. He also states that he is a diabetic. His vitals are as follows: HR 62, BP 155/95, RR 13, Temp. 37.2°C. He has diabetes mellitus, grade two cardiac heart failure, and general anxiety disorder. His BUN/Cr are 14/1.2. Which of the following medications is contraindicated given his past medical history?

A. A beta-blocker

B. An ACE inhibitor

C. An alpha-blocker

D. A diuretic

334. A 64-year-old male, being treated with antineo-plastic agents for acute myelogenous leukemia (and previously treated with bone marrow transplant), arrives in the ICU with a decreased level of consciousness that subsequently progresses to a comatose state. His oncologist relates to you that two days prior his mood began to change from pleasant and positive to placid and confused. He also began to report the perception of strange smells within his room, which others were unable to corroborate. Physical exam is significant for a temperature of 102.5°F and vesicular lesions present in various places on his torso and face. CSF demonstrates the presence of red blood cells.

How does the microbial agent responsible for this disease replicate its genome and assemble its component parts in the host?

A. It replicates its single-stranded DNA in the nucleus and is assembled in the cytoplasm.

B. It replicates its circular, double-stranded DNA in the nucleus and is assembled in the cytoplasm.

C. It replicates its linear, double-stranded DNA in the nucleus and is assembled in the nucleus.

D. It replicates its linear, double-stranded DNA in the cytoplasm using a DNA-dependent RNA polymerase and is assembled in the cytoplasm.

E. It replicates its circular, partially double-stranded DNA in the nucleus using a DNA polymerase with reverse transcriptase activity to synthesize an RNA intermediate, which is subsequently used to make the genomic DNA. The virus is assembled in the cytoplasm.

335. Cancer kills millions of people each year in the United States. Please select the appropriate answer with highest to lowest incidence:

A. Men: lungs, prostate, colon, melanoma

B. Women: breast, melanoma, colon, lungs

C. Men: prostate, lungs, colon, urinary tract

D. Women: lungs, breast, melanoma, colon

E. Men: lungs, colon, prostate, urinary tract

F. Women: lungs, breast, uterus, melanoma

336. A 63-year-old man presents to the primary care provider for his annual checkup. His past history reveals that he has been a cigarette smoker but gave up smoking five years prior to this visit. He drinks an occasional beer. His vital signs are: Temp. 37.5°C, RR 16, BP 135/85, Pulse 84. His height is 5'10" and his weight is 195 pounds. His physical exam was normal. What is the mean arterial pressure?

A. 50

B. 110

C. 102

D. 92

E. None of the above

337. A newborn infant who appeared healthy at birth began developing vomiting and lethargy during the first week of life. Physical exam revealed increased muscular tone and cerumen and urine that emitted a sweet odor. The urine was found to contain high levels of leucine, isoleucine, and valine. Which of the following enzymes is most likely defective in this patient?

A. Lactase

B. Phenylalanine hydroxylase

C. Aldolase B

D. Branched-chain alpha-ketoacid dehydrogenase

E. Glucose-6-phosphatase

338. You are sent to the emergency room to evaluate the mental status of a 30-year-old female who had been brought in following a suicide attempt. When you arrive at her bedside, you note she is wearing a bright orange hat and lots of makeup, is extremely friendly and flirtatious with the male staff, and does not appear depressed. On physical exam, you note multiple shallow knife incisions along the inside of both wrists, as well as several well-healed scars. This woman is most likely suffering from which disorder?

A. Paranoid personality disorder

B. Obsessive-compulsive personality disorder

C. Narcissistic personality disorder

D. Histrionic personality disorder

E. Schizotypal personality disorder

339. A 36-year-old woman presents to your medicine clinic with a history of amenorrhea, decreased peripheral vision, and a white secretion from her breasts. Which of the following findings are consistent with this clinical picture?

- **A.** Bitemporal hemianopia/decreased prolactin
- **B.** Central scotoma/decreased prolactin
- **C.** Homonymous hemianopia/increased prolactin
- **D.** Central scotoma/increased prolactin
- **E.** Bitemporal hemianopia/increased prolactin

340. A 22-year-old male college student comes to the clinic with a dry barking cough that does not want to leave. He states that the cough is worst at night. A chest x-ray shows an interstitial infiltrate. **(See Figure 340.)** Some of the others in his class have a similar cough. The patient most likely has:

- **A.** *Mycoplasma*
- **B.** *Legionella*
- **C.** *Chlamydia pneumoniae*
- **D.** *Coxiella burnetii*
- **E.** *Chlamydia psittaci*

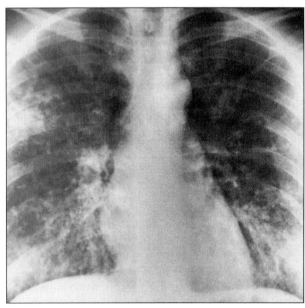

Figure 340   Reproduced with permission from Armstrong. Diagnostic Imaging. Blackwell Science, Inc., 2000.

341. Ms. Big is admitted to the hospital with atrial fibrillations. You want to rule out thyroid disease as a contributory factor for the arrhythmia. Which test is the single best diagnostic test for thyroid function?

- **A.** T_3
- **B.** T_4
- **C.** RT_3
- **D.** TSH
- **E.** TRH
- **F.** FT_4
- **G.** Thyroxine-binding globulin

342. A week after a heart attack, a 55-year-old man experiences shortness of breath, easy fatigue, and tiredness on exertion. On physical exam, he has weight gain, hepatomegaly, edema of lower extremities, and an S3 gallop. The right ventricle is enlarged based on EKG. What is the most likely abnormal parameter of the capillary fluid exchange?

- **A.** Decrease plasma protein
- **B.** Increase capillary permeability
- **C.** Increase capillary pressure
- **D.** Increase interstitial fluid colloid osmotic pressure
- **E.** None of the above

343. A 43-year-old white female, on oral contraceptives, obese and with a sedentary lifestyle, presents to the ER with leg pain. She has no shortness of breath, chest pain, or other complaint. Vital signs are normal. Physical exam is remarkable only for lower leg tenderness extending into the thigh on the left side. You order Doppler flow studies of her legs, which are positive for deep vein thrombosis. You immediately start regular heparin. Using the classic treatment of heparin and Coumadin, when should you start the Coumadin?

- **A.** Immediately
- **B.** 24 to 48 hours after beginning treatment with heparin
- **C.** Just before discharge, in two days
- **D.** In five days, then keep the patient in house until INR is two to three

344. After working a shift on labor and delivery, a fellow medical student comes up and asks you which of the following diseases is not routinely tested for on a routine screening of metabolic diseases of the newborn.

A. Phenylketonuria (PKU)
B. Hypothyroidism
C. Hypoparathyroidism
D. Biotinidase deficiency
E. Maple syrup urine disease

345. You enter an exam room to see a pediatric patient for a well-child exam. The child cries and clings to her mother as you approach. You are aware that the child is exhibiting normal developmental behavior. What is this called and what age is this child?

A. Rapprochement, age 12 to14 months
B. Rapprochement, age 16 to 24 months
C. Core gender identity, age 24 to 30 months
D. Stranger anxiety, age 16 to 20 months
E. Stranger anxiety, age 7 to 9 months

346. A young, healthy 25-year-old comes to your office for her yearly female examination. She would like to start taking combination oral contraceptives for birth control. Which of the following are potential side effects?

A. Edema
B. Decreased risk of myocardial infarction
C. Increased risk of endometrial cancer
D. Increased risk of ovarian cancer

347. A 9-year-old child from Colombia is brought to your office by his new adoptive parents. The child is below weight and height for age and is virtually blind on exam. Otherwise, the child's exam is unremarkable. Which vitamin deficiency is the likely culprit?

A. Vitamin A
B. Biotin
C. Vitamin C
D. Vitamin D
E. Vitamin E

348. An 8-year-old boy with pectus carinatum is brought to the clinic because his mother has noticed some bluish discoloration of his face and neck. His mother states that her son has no appetite, is prone to fevers, and does not want to play with his toys. On exam the child is pale, cyanotic, and answers only when asked a question. Physical examination shows positive distended neck veins, axillary and supraclavicular lymphadenopathy; cardiovascular exam shows: S1, S2, no S3, no S4, no murmurs. Pulmonary examination shows decreased breath sounds on the right lung base. You send him for a CT of the chest that shows mediastinal lymphadenopathy. Biopsy of the nodes is done and treatment is started right away. His mother asks you why her son continues to have the bluish discoloration on his face and neck. You explain that he has:

A. Eisenmenger's syndrome
B. Cardiomyopathy
C. Superior vena caval syndrome
D. COPD
E. Contusion due to a coagulopathy disorder

349. An 85-year-old man is brought in by his wife. She explains that he is having nausea, vomiting, and some visual changes. During the history, you find out that the patient has multiple medical problems including depression, congestive heart failure, BPH, and hypothyroidism. He was recently started on a "water pill." His other medications are "for my heart," "for my thyroid," "hormone for my prostate," and aspirin. Laboratory analysis shows a serum sodium of 142 mEq/L and potassium of 3.0 mEq/L. Which of the following drugs is most likely responsible for his symptoms?

A. Prozac (fluoxetine)
B. BuSpar (buspirone)
C. Digoxin
D. Proscar (finasteride)
E. Thyroxin

350. Recently, the World Congress of Medical Students elected you as the purveyor of new ideas. While preparing for your first assignment, you realize you need to find a derivative from a phospholipid that causes vasodilation, inhibits platelet aggregation, and increases the concentration of cAMP. You select:

A. Thromboxane A2
B. Prostaglandin E2
C. Prostaglandin I2
D. Leukotriene E4
E. Leukotriene B4

BLOCK VII - ANSWER KEY

301-C	314-A	327-A	339-E
302-E	315-C	328-A	340-A
303-A	316-A	329-C	341-D
304-B	317-B	330-A	342-C
305-C	318-D	331-B	343-B
306-B	319-D	332-B	344-C
307-E	320-A	333-A	345-E
308-E	321-A	334-C	346-A
309-E	322-E	335-C	347-A
310-D	323-E	336-C	348-C
311-A	324-C	337-D	349-D
312-B	325-C	338-D	350-C
313-B	326-B		

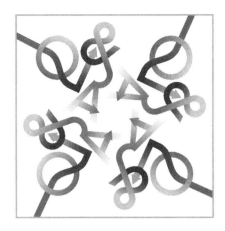

ANSWERS
BLOCK 7

301. C This patient presents with the clinical features of deep venous thrombosis (DVT), requiring anticoagulant therapy. Heparin directly stimulates the activity of antithrombin III. In turn, antithrombin III inhibits the activity of thrombin, thus preventing the conversion of fibrinogen into fibrin. This allows the body's own fibrinolytic forces to act on the existing fibrin clot causing the DVT without any further worsening from new clot formation. Antithrombin III also acts to inhibit Factor XIIa, Factor IXa, and Factor Xa.

A. Plasmin stimulates the hydrolysis of the hard fibrin clot but is not acted upon by heparin.
B. Plasminogen is converted to plasmin by anticoagulants such as streptokinase and tPA, but heparin does not act upon it.
D. Prothrombin (Factor II) is not acted upon by heparin. It is a precursor to thrombin.
E. Factor VII is part of the extrinsic pathway and is stimulated by vitamin K, and thus inhibited by warfarin, but it is not acted upon by heparin.

302. E This patient displays symptoms of schizophrenia, most likely of the paranoid type. The most appropriate medication for this patient would be an antipsychotic. Clozapine is the only medication in the list that falls under this category.

A. Sertraline is an antidepressant medication.
B. Methylphenidate is a psychostimulant, often used in the treatment of ADHD.
C. Lithium is a mood stabilizer, often used in the treatment of bipolar disorder.
D. Citalopram is an antidepressant medication.

303. A This patient has received a *Staphylococcus aureus* infection from the stab wound to the abdomen. This became apparent when the patient became febrile and septic from the gram-positive and coagulase-positive bacteria. This bacteria can also cause food poisoning.

B. *Staphylococcus epidermidis* is most commonly associated with prosthetic and shunt infections.
C. *Streptococcus pyogenes* is most commonly associated with scarlet fever.
D. A major cause of meningitis is *Neisseria meningitidis*.
E. A leading cause of STD is *Neisseria gonorrhoeae*.

304. B Antimicrobials that are protein synthesis inhibitors are classified as bacteriostatic or bactericidal depending on their mechanism of action. Bacteriostatic drugs arrest growth and development of bacteria, leaving the total number of viable organisms the same. Bactericidal drugs work in such a way as to kill the bacteria, thus decreasing the total number of bacteria. Tobramycin is an aminoglycoside used to treat serious gram-negative infections such as *Pseudomonas*.

A, **C**, **D**, and **E** are all bacteriostatic.

305. C The ulnar nerve is responsible for sensation in the medial $1^1/_2$ fingers as well as the following muscles: flexor carpi ulnaris, flexor digitorum profundus, adductor pollicis, 8 interossei, 3 hypothenar, and lumbricals in the fourth and fifth fingers.

A. The musculocutaneous nerve innervates mostly the forearm flexors and medial forearm.
B. The median nerve's motor control is the wrist flexors. The lateral $3^1/_2$ fingers on the palmar side are also under sensory control of the median nerve.
D. The radial nerve innervates the wrist extensors and forearm extensors. It is also responsible for sensation of the lateral $3^1/_2$ fingers on the dorsal side.
E. The long thoracic nerve innervates the serratus anterior muscle. A lesion leads to winging of the scapula.

306. B Infectious mononucleosis, usually caused by the Epstein-Barr virus, best fits the description above. EBV is a herpesvirus transmitted through saliva; mono usually presents with fatigue, anorexia, sore throat, and lymphadenopathy in young adults or adolescents. The pharyngitis is frequently associated with a white exudate. Patients with mono who are given amoxicillin will develop a rash 90% of the time.

A. The presentation is classic for mono. Although HIV may present in this manner (especially at time of seroconversion), the rash with Amoxil makes mono the correct answer.

C. The presentation is more consistent with mono.

D. Incorrect because of the reaction to the amoxicillin. The presentations for mono and streptococcal pharyngitis are very similar (almost identical) and can be differentiated for certain on the basis of cultures and blood tests.

E. Incorrect for the same reason as C.

307. E Diagnostic testing for sickle cell anemia involves detection of the defective hemoglobin (HbS). This is done through gel electrophoresis.

A. PCR is used to amplify a gene sequence of interest for detection using a variation of gel electrophoresis known as Southern blotting. PCR testing is effective in testing for viral genes (HIV).

B. Betke-Kleihauer acid elution is a test used for Rh incompatibility following delivery by treating a maternal blood sample with an acidic solution that discolors fetal red blood cells in contrast to maternal red blood cells. This test is not applicable in sickle cell patients.

C. X-ray crystallography is used to identify protein structures but is very difficult to pursue as a routine diagnostic test for sickle cell anemia.

D. Sanger DNA chain termination method is used to determine the DNA sequence of a gene of interest. This test involves the use of radioactive labeling to known DNA bases that are then paired to their nonradioactive counterparts. This can then be used to determine a gene sequence of interest.

308. E Nafcillin is effective against *Staph aureus* that is sensitive to methicillin and it is excreted primarily through the liver instead of through the kidney.

A. Ampicillin is not effective against penicillin G–resistant *Staph aureus*.

B. Ticarcillin is not effective against penicillin G–resistant *Staph aureus* but was instead designed to combat gram-negative organisms.

C. Penicillin V has no significant difference in its coverage as compared to penicillin G.

D. Although oxacillin would be effective against this organism, it is primarily processed through the kidneys.

309. E In cardiac tamponade there is no y-wave descent and a prominent x-wave descent. The y-descent represents the beginning of diastole when blood flows passively into the ventricle through the tricuspid valve, representing ventricular filling. The cardiac tamponade in this case is due to myocardial injury from blunt trauma to the chest. Each time the heart contracts, the pericardial sac fills with blood, preventing the heart from relaxing properly. The next contraction is not as effective as the previous one, and further blood accumulation worsens relaxation. The volume capacity of the four chambers of the heart becomes fixed. The ejection phase is the only time that blood can enter the heart, so that when blood leaves the ventricles, the veins transmit blood into the atria. This is reflected in the steep x-descent. Normally, the y-descent reflects blood moving from the atria into the ventricle, but since the volume is static, it simply equilibrates when the AV valves open and thus there is no y-descent. Clinically this is reflected in a narrowing of the pulse pressure, jugular venous distention, and muffled heart sounds.

A. The a-wave represents atrial contraction and would be absent in atrial fibrillation or have increased amplitude in mitral stenosis.

B. The c-wave represents right ventricular contraction with the tricuspid valve bulging into the atrium. This is not significantly affected in cardiac tamponade.

C. The t-wave is part of the EKG representing electrical, not mechanical, activity of the heart. It is not part of the jugular venous pulse.

D. The v-wave is typically what produces the visible characteristics of the jugular venous pulse. It is typically accentuated in mitral insufficiency.

310. D The following factors increase the affinity of hemoglobin for oxygen: decreased PCO_2, increased pH, decreased temperature, and decreased 2,3-DPG concentration. In carbon monoxide poisoning, the affinity of hemoglobin for carbon monoxide is much higher than its affinity for oxygen. Therefore, the affinity of hemoglobin for the remaining oxygen sites is much higher, inhibiting the ability of the body to unload oxygen in the tissues. Fetal hemoglobin, or hemoglobin F, does not bind 2,3-DPG as tightly as adult hemoglobin, therefore increasing its affinity for oxygen.

The following factors decrease the affinity of hemoglobin for oxygen: increased PCO_2, decreased pH, increased temperature, and increased 2,3-DPG. With exercise, the working tissue produces more CO_2, therefore reducing tissue pH and encouraging oxygen delivery to the muscle. Exercise also increases temperature.

A. When the metabolic activity of tissue is decreased (i.e., skeletal muscle at rest), temperature is decreased, and this leads to increased affinity of hemoglobin for oxygen. Therefore, less oxygen is unloaded into resting muscle versus exercising skeletal muscle.

B. 2,3-DPG is a by-product of glycolysis, which binds hemoglobin and decreases its affinity for oxygen. This facilitates the unloading of oxygen into tissue. Therefore, decreased 2,3-DPG concentrations would lead to increased affinity of hemoglobin.

C. Hemoglobin F leads to increased affinity of hemoglobin for oxygen as explained above.

E. Carbon monoxide poisoning leads to increased affinity of hemoglobin for oxygen as explained above.

311. A CK-MB is the earliest and most sensitive detectable enzyme that rises in acute myocardial infarction in the early stages (within 3 to 12 hours). However, one should be aware of the limitations of this enzyme as an early indicator, which may be sensitive but not specific as conditions other than a myocardial infarction can elevate CK-MB (i.e., myocarditis, pericarditis, etc.). Other laboratory findings (nonspecific) indicating an acute myocardial infarction include an elevated erythrocyte sedimentation rate and leukocytosis.

B. CK-BB is found predominantly in the brain.

C. CK-MM is found predominantly in muscle; however, it can be elevated in conditions where destruction of muscle has taken place to release amounts of CK-MM into the circulation.

D. LDH can be used in the detection of a myocardial infarction; however, this is only detectable 12 hours following an MI, and will remain elevated for an additional 10 to 14 days after infarction. Since this question asks for the most immediately detectable test, the CK-MB would offer more immediate results.

312. B Herpes simplex virus (HSV) is an enveloped, double-stranded DNA virus. The herpesvirus and poxvirus families are enveloped, double-stranded DNA viruses with linear genomes. The hepadnavirus family is also enveloped, and primarily double-stranded DNA with a circular genome.

A. There are no enveloped, single-stranded DNA virus families.

C. The hepadnaviruses are enveloped DNA viruses that have a circular genome, which is double-stranded for most of its length but does contain a single-stranded region as well.

D. The only nonenveloped, single-stranded DNA virus family is the parvoviruses.

E. The nonenveloped, double-stranded DNA viruses are the papovavirus and the adenovirus families.

F. The enveloped, positive-strand RNA viruses that replicate via a DNA intermediate are the retroviruses, such as HIV.

313. B The first branch of the external carotid artery is the superior thyroid artery and thus would be the artery nearest to the obstruction.

A. The inferior thyroid artery arises from the subclavian artery.

C. The lingual artery branches from the external carotid after the superior thyroid artery.

D. The vertebral artery arises from the subclavian artery.

E. The facial artery arises from the external carotid distal to the superior thyroid artery.

314. A Malignant hyperthermia represents a potentially fatal adverse reaction to drugs used for anesthesia, but can be effectively treated with dantrolene if it is recognized quickly. The condition is hereditary and presents with a rapid rise in body temperature and muscle rigidity. Surgery should be stopped immediately, cooling of the body begun, acid-base and electrolyte imbalances corrected, oxygen provided and large amounts of dantrolene infused.

B. Succinylcholine is one of the drugs that may trigger malignant hyperthermia.

C. Propranolol is not the correct treatment.

D. Acetaminophen is not the correct answer. While it is an effective antipyretic, it is not the treatment for malignant hyperthermia.

E. Inhaled anesthetic agents such as halothane may trigger malignant hyperthermia.

315. C Intrinsic factor is produced by parietal cells of the gastric glands and is required for absorption of vitamin B12 in the terminal ileum. In chronic atrophic gastritis, intrinsic factor is not produced, leading to vitamin B12 deficiency, megaloblastic anemia, and neurologic sequelae. The patient's fatigue is likely related to his anemia, and parenteral vitamin B12 replacement is required to prevent neurologic sequelae.

A. Although folic acid deficiency is another important cause of megaloblastic anemia, it is not likely to be present in a patient with a diet including leafy green vegetables.

B. Niacin deficiency is characterized by dermatitis, diarrhea, and dementia.

D. Vitamin C deficiency results in scurvy, characterized by easy bruising and bleeding gums.

316. A This is a description of an infant with Tay-Sachs disease, one of the lysosomal storage disorders. This autosomal recessive disease is common in Ashkenazi Jews, and is caused by a total lack of hexosaminidase A. The infantile form of this disease is a uniformly fatal neurodegenerative disease.

B. The function of mitochondria is normal in Tay-Sachs disease.

C. Protein synthesis is normal in Tay-Sachs disease.

D. Nuclear transcription of DNA to mRNA is normal in Tay-Sachs disease.

317. B Antisocial personality disorder (ASPD), more common in men, is a pervasive pattern of inability to conform to society's norms. Diagnosis requires that problems exist since age 15, and evidence of conduct disorder prior to age 15. Although these individuals may appear as charming or slick, their underlying character is one of manipulation, legal problems, cons, impulsivity, and aggressiveness; perhaps the most striking is the lack of remorse they feel for their unacceptable actions.

A. Malingering is when patients fake an illness or symptoms in order to get some gain (usually financial or getting out of jail).

C. Dependent personality disorder is diagnosed in individuals with a pervasive pattern of relying excessively on others for decisions and support.

D. Conversion disorder presents with significant neurologic complaints (not able to walk, numbness) but there is no clinical explanation for the symptoms.

E. Conduct disorder is the "child version" of ASPD but would not be diagnosed after age 18.

318. D Blood levels of medications decrease by 50% during each half-life. The half-life of this medication is 1.3 days. After 3.9 days, or three half-lives, the plasma level would be 1.125 mg/L, which is within the therapeutic range of 1–1.5 mg/L.

A. The plasma level would not decrease if the medication were not withheld.

B. After 1.3 days, which is one half-life, the plasma level would be 4.5 mg/L.

C. After 2.6 days, which is two half-lives, the plasma level would be 2.25 mg/L.

E. After 5.2 days, which is four half-lives, the plasma level would be 0.5625 mg/L.

319. D Parathyroid related peptide (PTRP) is frequently produced by squamous cell cancers, leading to increased serum levels of calcium. In fact, hypercalcemia is the most common paraneoplastic syndrome found with lung squamous cell cancers.

A. Small cell cancers metastasize earlier than squamous cell cancers; small cell cancers have already usually spread by the time they are discovered.

B. Squamous cell cancers tend to develop centrally and then spread peripherally.

C. This cancer frequently metastasizes to the liver, bones, and brain.

E. Kulchitsky cells, a type of neuroendocrine cell, may develop into carcinoid tumors, not squamous cell cancers.

320. A The autonomic nervous system helps control smooth muscle, cardiac muscle, and a variety of glands (lacrimal, submandibular, sublingual, and parotid). During the start response (half of the fight-or-flight), the ANS responds by increasing sympathetic tone. In this case, the results are dilation of the pupils, increased heart rate, decreased gastrointestinal blood flow, and dilation of the bronchial tubes.

B. The pupils and the bronchial tubes dilate.
C. The pupils dilate and the blood flow to the gastrointestinal tract is decreased.
D. The heart rate is increased, the blood flow to the gastrointestinal tract is decreased and the bronchial tubes dilate.
E. The pupils dilate, the heart rate increases, and the blood flow to the gastrointestinal tract is decreased.

321. A Patients with Conn's syndrome often present with weakness, headaches, and new-onset hypertension. Hypersecretion of aldosterone, usually by an adrenal adenoma, leads to increased sodium absorption with concomitant loss of potassium.

B. Although Cushing's syndrome can cause fatigue and hypertension, it is characterized by alterations in body habitus, including central obesity, hirsutism, and abdominal striae.
C. Addison's disease causes weakness, hypotension, and often increased skin pigmentation.
D. High salt intake would not cause these symptoms or electrolyte abnormalities.

322. E This patient has a history of recurrent UTIs and now has developed what appears to be a struvite stone, which tend to be large. A struvite stone is made up of magnesium ammonium phosphate crystals. They are associated with bacteria that produce urease, such as *Proteus mirabilis*.

A. About 80% of community-acquired UTIs are caused by *E. coli*. This would be the suspected organism in a woman with a UTI were it not for the complicating struvite stone.
B. This organism is a common cause of UTIs in catheterized patients. It is also not associated with struvite stones.
C. *Staphylococcus aureus* is not a common cause of UTIs.
D. *K. pneumoniae* is another gram-negative bacteria causing UTIs, but like *E. coli* does not produce struvite stones.

323. E The patient in this case likely has hypokalemia, judging from the characteristic EKG findings and weakness. Furosemide is a loop diuretic that is sometimes used for hypertension refractory to thiazide diuretics. Its serious side effects include sodium and water retention and potassium wasting.

A. Monopril is an ACE inhibitor that is used for hypertension, among other conditions. Like all ACE inhibitors, it decreases aldosterone levels. Aldosterone is responsible for retaining sodium and excreting potassium. When it is reduced, potassium is retained and hyperkalemia may result.
B. Spironolactone is an aldosterone receptor antagonist. Thus, it has a similar effect to ACE inhibitors and can cause hyperkalemia, not hypokalemia.
C. Amiloride is a potassium-sparing diuretic that acts at the distal convoluted tubule. It doesn't cause potassium wasting like furosemide, and can result in hyperkalemia.
D. Irbesartan is an angiotensin receptor blocker. By blocking angiotensin, it reduces aldosterone (which is released from the adrenals by angiotensin II). Thus, potassium is retained.

324. C This is a classic presentation of diabetic ketoacidosis, which commonly occurs when patients with type I diabetes mellitus fail to take insulin or have increased insulin requirements due to infection. Decreased insulin and elevated glucagon levels cause the release of fatty acids, which are subsequently converted to the ketone bodies acetoacetate and β-hydroxybutyrate.

A. Ascorbic acid (vitamin C) would not be expected to be present in high concentrations in diabetic ketoacidosis.
B. Folic acid levels are unaffected in diabetic ketoacidosis.
D. Oxaloacetate, an intermediary of the TCA cycle, is not elevated in diabetic ketoacidosis.

325. C Prevalence is the number of cases in the population at a given time; incidence is the number of new cases in the population over a certain length of time (usually one year). Prevalence is equal to length of the disease process multiplied by the incidence (assumes both are stable). Prevalence is greater than incidence in conditions such as diabetes, which are more long-term or chronic.

A, B, D, E. Due to the limited nature of this illness, the number of cases at any given time (prevalence) would not likely exceed the number of new cases developing over a year.

326. B The peroneal nerve (L4-S4) is responsible for the tibialis anterior, extensor hallicus longus, and extensor digitorum longus muscles. Damage to the nerve results in an inability to evert the foot and dorsiflex the ankle and toe.

A. The disease process described here is Legg-Calve-Perthes disease, which is avascular necrosis of the femoral head. The incidence is higher in boys than in girls. Patients with LCP disease have an insidious onset of hip or groin pain and present with a limp. The girl in this case has no complaints related to the hip or groin. The treatment is either surgery or casting.

C. The tibial nerve (L4-L3) is responsible for foot inversion, ankle flexion, and ankle jerk. In our patient, the ankle jerk is intact and inversion is intact.

D. The disease process described here is spina bifida, which is a defect in the development of the dorsal vertebral arches. Typically, children with neurological sequelae present earlier than 8 years old. In addition, spina bifida patients will commonly have bilateral involvement. During pregnancy, mothers will often have increased alpha-fetoprotein levels and decreased intake of folic acid during the organogenesis period (second through eighth weeks).

E. Tissue swelling and inflammation are also called sprains. Sprains typically subside after three to five days of rest and without neurological sequelae.

327. A Procainamide is a class IA antiarrhythmic, and is used to convert atrial fibrillation to sinus rhythm when electroversion is not indicated or not preferred.

B. Atenolol is a beta-blocker and is used in atrial fibrillation for rate control, but will not convert the patient back to sinus rhythm.

C. Diltiazem is also used for rate control, but should not be used in patients with CHF, as it has a negative inotropic effect.

D. Digoxin can also be used for rate control as it blocks AV node conduction. It can also be used in CHF because it is a positive inotrope. However, it will not convert a patient in atrial fibrillation to a normal sinus rhythm.

E. Verapamil is a calcium channel blocker like diltiazem, and can be used only for rate control, not conversion to a normal sinus rhythm.

328. A The patient described likely has xeroderma pigmentosum, a disease caused by inherited defects in recognition of DNA damage caused by ultraviolet light or in nucleotide excision and repair. Clinically, xeroderma pigmentosum is characterized by extraordinary photosensitivity and malignant skin tumors in sun-exposed areas, as well as freckles, telangiectases, papillomas, keratoses, and keratitic changes and/or tumors on the eyelids and cornea.

B. The immune system is normal in xeroderma pigmentosum.

C. Tyrosinase is deficient in albinism, characterized by very light-colored skin, hair, and eyes.

D. HGPRT is deficient in Lesch-Nyhan syndrome, which causes mental retardation and self-mutilation.

329. C While all of the above species can be found in the mouth, the correct answer is *Actinomyces israelii*. This anaerobic actinomycete is located in the intragingival crevices, sharing the normal flora of the mouth with *Bacteroides*, *Fusobacterium*, *Clostridium*, and *Peptostreptococcus*, all of which can cause lung abscesses. Actinomyces are known for slow-developing jaw infections in patients who are debilitated or have poor dental hygiene. These patients may also develop concomitantly lung and abdominal abscesses. Treatment for *Actinomyces* infection is penicillin G with surgical drainage of the abscess.

A. *Strep mutans* is a member of the viridans group making up one-half of normal mouth flora. This species produces dental plaque, but is not a common cause of dental, jaw, or disseminated infections.

B, D, and E are incorrect. *Eikenella* is commonly seen in association with human bite wounds. However, it does not cause jaw and lung infections, and neither does the *Candida* group. While *Staph* infection could produce lung abscesses, it is an uncommon cause of the combination of infections described here

330. A Variant angina (Prinzmetal's angina) occurs at rest in atypical patterns such as after exercise or nocturnally. The angina is caused by coronary spasm and is associated with ST elevation on EKG during symptoms. When the vessel constricts, the resistance increases and can lead to distress if perfusion is compromised. Resistance is directly proportional to viscosity and inversely proportional to the radius to the fourth power, and the formula is:

$$\text{Resistance} = \frac{8(\text{viscosity}) \times \text{length}}{\Pi r^4}$$

B and **C.** Incorrect.

D, E, and **F.** Incorrect. Vessel dilatation would cause a decrease in resistance.

331. B Tays-Sachs disease is an autosomal recessive disease, caused by a deficiency in the enzyme hexosaminidase A. There is a lysosomal accumulation of gangliosides.

A. Alpha-1,4-glucosidase is deficient in Pompe disease, resulting in the accumulation of glycogen within the lysosomes.
C. Alpha-galactosidase A is deficient in Fabry disease, resulting in the accumulation of ceramide trihexoside within the lysosomes.
D. Sphingomyelinase is deficient in Niemann-Pick disease, resulting in the accumulation of sphingomyelin within the lysosomes.
E. Arylsulfatase A is deficient in metachromatic leukodystrophy resulting in the accumulation of sulfatide within the lysosomes.

332. B Enuresis (bed-wetting) occurs during stage 3-4 or slow-wave sleep, and is characterized by the presence of delta waves. Delta waves are high voltage (amplitude) and low frequency.

A. Sleep spindles and K complexes are most characteristic of stage 2 sleep.
C. Beta waves with sawtooth appearance are most characteristic of REM sleep. Beta waves are low voltage, high frequency.
D. Theta waves are most characteristic of stage 1 sleep.
E. Alpha waves are most characteristic of when a person is awake, but relaxed with eyes closed.

333. A There is a lot of extra information in this question. What you should focus on is that his heart rate is pretty low as it is. If you give him a beta-blocker, his pulse may fall below 60. Also, a beta-blocker may worsen his CHF, although recently this view has been challenged.

B. ACE inhibitor would help his HTN and protect his kidneys.
C. In high amounts, they may act as a beta-blocker as well, but clearly, the best answer is A.
D. A diuretic would reduce his HTN and CHF.

334. C This patient is immunocompromised due to his ongoing treatment designed to destroy the leukemic cell line. As a result, he is at risk for a number of opportunistic infections. The signs and symptoms given here, though, should lead you to place herpes encephalitis high upon the differential. Confusion and coma indicate that some process is affecting the brain, most likely infectious given his immunocompromised state. Mood changes and olfactory hallucinations, as described in the case, indicate temporal lobe involvement. There is only one viral infection that affects the temporal lobes of the brain, that being herpes simplex virus (HSV). Specifically, HSV-1 is associated with hemorrhagic encephalitis of the temporal lobes. Hemorrhage is indicated by the presence of RBCs in the CSF. The presence of vesicular lesions on the body further leads in the direction of some virus from the Herpesviridae family. Every virus in the Herpesviridae family (HSV, VZV, EBV, CMV) replicates its DNA and assembles its component parts in the nucleus.

A. This describes the characteristics and method of replication and propagation utilized by the Parvoviridae family.
B. This describes the characteristics and method of replication and propagation utilized by the Papovaviridae family.
D. This describes the characteristics and method of replication and propagation utilized by the Poxviridae family.
E. This describes the characteristics and method of replication and propagation utilized by the Hepadnaviridae family (responsible for hepatitis B).

335. C Prostate cancer is the cancer with highest incidence in males. Yet, most men with prostate cancer die of unrelated causes. Essentially, every male who lives long enough will get prostate cancer. Prostate cancer tends to spread to the spine and cause pathologic fractures.

A. Lung cancer is the number one killer in both men and women, but the question is asking about incidence, not mortality.
B. Both colon cancer and lung cancer are more common than melanoma in both sexes.
D. Although lung cancer kills more women, breast cancer is more common.
E and **F.** See above.

336. C Mean arterial pressure is calculated as follows:

MAP = diastolic pressure + 1/3 pulse pressure

Pulse pressure = systolic pressure − diastolic pressure

A. Incorrect. 50 is the pulse pressure.
B and **D.** Incorrect.
E. Incorrect.

337. D Maple syrup urine disease is due to a defect in the ability to degrade branched amino acids (leucine, isoleucine, and valine). Symptoms usually manifest in the first week of life and can include neurological defects or death. Patients must be dialyzed and put on lifelong dietary restriction to minimize levels of these amino acids.

A. Lactase deficiency is associated with bloating and cramps after milk consumption and usually manifests later in life.
B. Phenylalanine hydroxylase deficiency results in phenylketonuria.
C. Aldolase B deficiency results in hypoglycemia and toxicity secondary to rapid accumulation of fructose-1-phosphate. Patients usually are asymptomatic until their diets are switched from milk to foods containing fructose or sucrose, such as fruit, fruit juice, or sweetened cereal.
E. Glucose-6-phosphate deficiency (Von Gierke's disease) results in an inability to degrade glycogen and is characterized by severe fasting hypoglycemia and increased glycogen found in the liver.

338. D Histrionic belongs to the cluster B group of personality disorders. Histrionic individuals are more often women and tend to be overly dramatic, attention seeking, and sexually provocative. In this situation, the patient is using mock suicide attempts, as noted by the shallow knife wounds, to gain attention.

A. Paranoid belongs to the cluster A group of personality disorders. Paranoid individuals tend to be distrustful and suspicious of others and utilize projection as an ego defense.
B. Obsessive-compulsive belongs to the cluster C group of personality disorders. Individuals suffering from obsessive-compulsive personality disorder are perfectionists, desiring control and order.
C. Narcissistic belongs to the cluster B group of personality disorders. Narcissistic individuals tend to be pompous and display a sense of entitlement, expecting that they deserve the "best" of everything.

E. Schizotypal belongs to the cluster A group of personality disorders. Schizotypal individuals display magical thinking (i.e., the belief that their thoughts can control the course of events), odd thought patterns and appearance, but are not necessarily psychotic.

339. E The patient has a pituitary adenoma, which presents as a bitemporal hemianopia with endocrine abnormalities. The visual field defect is the lateral half of the visual field in both eyes. The bitemporal hemianopia is a result of pressure on the optic chiasm. In these patients, the prolactin is often elevated with galactorrhea and amenorrhea. Other signs include headache, acromegaly, and blurred vision.

A. The prolactin will be increased.
B. A central scotoma is usually caused by inflammation of the optic disc. The prolactin would be increased.
C. A lesion of the left optic tract causes a homonymous hemianopia.
D. A central scotoma is usually caused by inflammation of the optic disc, which is not consistent with this clinical picture.

340. A This is likely to be *Mycoplasma* pneumonia. This is quite common in young adults, especially where crowded conditions such as classrooms make droplet spread easier. It is transmitted through respiratory droplets. Sputum is scanty. Serum cold agglutinins are usually elevated.

B. This type of atypical pneumonia is seen in alcoholics, diabetic patients, or those exposed to contaminated air conditioning. There is no person-to-person transmission.
C. This is primarily seen in elderly patients. They present with a sore throat and hoarseness of the voice.
D. *Coxiella burnetii* is associated with farm animals.
E. *Chlamydia psittaci* is found in parrot or turkey feces.

341. D Most clinicians and laboratory pathologists agree that TSH is the single best indicator of thyroid function. Our bodies regulate TSH levels such that most euthyroid individuals have TSH levels in a very narrow range.

A. T_3 is almost never used in clinical medicine.
B. Total T_4 used to be measured in the past. With current technology, we can measure free T_4.

C. Only in extreme rare cases would an rT_3 be of any value.

E. Thyroid releasing hormone is almost never measured. Tumors/adenomas producing excess TSH/TRH are extremely rare, with fewer than 10 reported cases in the literature.

F. FT_4 may be used if TSH level is not conclusive.

G. The body regulates free thyroid hormone and TSH. An increase or decrease of thyroxine-binding globulin usually does not lead to clinical hypo- or hyperthyroidism.

342. C Right-sided congestive heart failure is caused by pulmonary hypertension and left-sided heart failure. The congestion of the venous system affects the liver, kidneys, brain, pleural space, and interstitial tissues. The increased capillary pressure is due to the venous congestion of right-sided heart failure. The increased capillary pressure causes more fluid to move out of the vascular system. The filtration pressure is calculated as follows:

Filtration pressure =
[(Capillary pressure – interstitial fluid pressure) – (plasma colloid osmotic pressure – interstitial fluid colloid osmotic pressure)]

A. Decreased plasma protein occurs in patients with nephrotic syndrome and liver failure, and edema occurs in these patients because of decreased plasma colloid.

B. Increased capillary permeability occurs in burn patients, toxin ingestions, and infections. The inflammatory process causes leakage of the capillary membrane, allowing fluid to move out of the vascular system.

D. Interstitial fluid usually returns to the vascular system through the lymphatic system. Lymphatic blockage causes retention of both proteins/solutes and fluid to cause edema.

E. Incorrect.

343. B The teaching is that there is a paradoxical effect with the first dose of Coumadin. Having the heparin in the system for one to two days is thought to lessen this adverse effect. Modern treatment options include low-molecular-weight heparin, which can be easily dosed and does not require as close monitoring as does the PT INR when a patient is on long-term Coumadin.

A. As stated above, you would want to avoid the paradoxical effects of Coumadin.

C. The patient has to remain in the hospital to receive heparin and stabilize INR on Coumadin.

D. Neither the patient nor the insurance company is willing to wait this long for treatment.

344. C The level of parathyroid is not typically tested in newborns; there is no screening test for this problem in newborns.

A. Phenylketonuria is important to diagnose at birth due to the irreversible effects on intellectual development. If patients with PKU are not diagnosed early, the manifestations include pigmentation less than what would be expected by parents' level of pigmentation (dilute pigmentation), seizures, rash, and mental retardation.

B. Hypothyroidism is often suggested by the signs and symptoms at birth, which include macroglossia, lethargy, abdominal distention, hypothermia, respiratory distress, and hypotonia. If not treated early, it will result in mental retardation and dwarfism (cretinism).

D. Biotinidase deficiency causes developmental delay, alopecia, ataxia, and conjunctivitis.

E. Maple syrup urine disease left undiagnosed and untreated in the neonatal period can lead to seizures and death. MSUD or branched-chain ketoaciduria affects the amino acids leucine, isoleucine, and valine by failure of the branched-chain ketoacid decarboxylase enzyme.

345. E Stranger anxiety usually occurs between 7 and 9 months of age. Infants at this age are able to distinguish familiar faces from unfamiliar ones.

A. Rapprochement refers to the period when infants move away from a familiar caregiver and return for comfort. This occurs usually at age 16 to 24 months.

B. Rapprochement refers to the period when infants move away from a familiar caregiver and return for comfort.

C. Core gender identity refers to the infant's identification of himself or herself as male or female. This occurs between 18 and 30 months of age.

D. Stranger anxiety occurs between 7 to 9 months of age.

346. A Edema is a major side effect of oral contraceptives. There is also an increased risk of myocardial infarction. Other more common side effects are depression and headache.

B. There is an increased risk of myocardial infarction in women taking oral contraceptives.

C. There is a decreased risk of endometrial cancer in women taking oral contraceptives.

D. There is a decreased risk of ovarian cancer in women taking oral contraceptives.

347. A Vitamin A is a fat-soluble vitamin responsible for the major family of molecules known as the retinoids, which are vital for normal vision, reproduction, and growth. A deficiency in vitamin A initially leads to night blindness and eventually to xerophthalmia, severe dryness of the eye. Vitamin A deficiency is also far more common in tropical third-world countries than in industrialized nations.

B. Biotin deficiency is very unlikely because of the wide distribution of biotin in food and the manufacture of biotin by intestinal bacteria.

C. Vitamin C deficiency causes scurvy, which is manifested through defects in collagen hydroxylation. The result is swollen joints, anemia, dental abnormalities, weakened blood vessels, bleeding gums, and poor wound healing.

D. Vitamin D comes in a variety of forms and plays an essential role in the calcium and phosphate physiology in the body. A deficiency results in rickets, which causes skeletal deformities and alterations in growth.

E. A deficiency in vitamin E is vary rare and usually only occurs in premature infants and adults with lipid disorders.

348. C This patient has lymphoma with enlarged mediastinal lymph nodes and superior vena caval syndrome due to the compression of the vena cava by the large mediastinal lymph nodes. This in return decreases the flow of venous blood back to the heart and causes a pooling of venous blood in the head, neck, and upper extremities depending on the severity of blockage; hence the dusky cyanosis that is seen in patients.

A. This is seen in children who have congenital heart defects, atrial septal defect, ventricular septal defect, or patent ductus arteriosus that cause the normal left to right shunt to reverse to right to left causing more deoxygenated blood to be released into the circulation.

B. A cardiomyopathy would cause peripheral cyanosis, not just head and neck cyanosis.

D. Chronic obstructive pulmonary disease is seen in adults due to restrictive lung disease from an insult. Patients present with pursed lips, barrel chest, or "blue bloater."

E. If this child had a coagulopathy disorder he would have petechiae and/or ecchymoses, not cyanosis.

349. D This is a case of digoxin toxicity. Because of the new diuretic, most likely a thiazide, the patient has become hypokalemic, which can induce digoxin toxicity. This can also happen with the loop diuretics such as furosemide. It is a common side effect and since both medications may be used for CHF, you should be aware of this interaction/side effect.

A. Prozac is an SSRI. Most common side effects of most SSRIs are reduced sexual desire and appetite and sleep changes. In extremely rare cases they may cause hyponatremia.

B. BuSpar is used for patients with anxiety. It has no effect on electrolytes.

C. Proscar (finasteride) inhibits 5-alpha-reductase, which inhibits the conversion of testosterone to DHT, 5-alpha-dihydrotestosterone. It is used to treat benign prostatic hypertrophy (BPH). Its side effects are largely related to sexual function and include impotence.

E. Too much thyroxin presents as thyroid storm or hyperthyroidism.

350. C Prostacyclin or prostaglandin I2 is produced by vascular endothelium to vasodilate, inhibit platelet aggregation, and increase the concentration of cAMP.

A. Thromboxane A2 is produced by platelets to promote platelet aggregation, vasoconstrict, decrease formation of cAMP, and contract smooth muscle.

B. Prostaglandin E2 is produced throughout the body and primarily acts as a vasodilator without affecting the platelet system.

D. Leukotriene E4 is an end product of leukotriene synthesis and causes vasoconstriction and bronchoconstriction.

E. Leukotriene B4 increases chemotaxis of neutrophils.

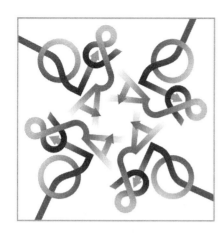

INDEX